To Alison, Emma, Robert and Katie and Julie,
Martha and Fergus with all our love

Essentials of
Paediatric Intensive Care

C G Stack, FRCA
Director of Intensive Care
Sheffield Children's Hospital

P Dobbs, FRCA
Consultant Anaesthetist
Royal Hallamshire Hospital, Sheffield

www.greenwich-medical.co.uk

© 2004
Greenwich Medical Media Limited
137 Euston Road
London
NW1 2AA

870 Market St, Ste 720
San Francisco, CA 94102

ISBN 1 84110 053 6

First Published 2004

A catalogue record for this book is available from the British Library

Typeset by Mizpah Publishing Services, Chennai, India

Printed in Malta by the Gutenberg Press Ltd

Distributed by Plymbridge Distributors Ltd
and in the USA by JAMCO Distribution

CONTENTS

PREFACE

The aim of this book is to be a practical handbook providing easily accessible information for medical and nursing staff who are involved in looking after sick children. It is aimed at those who work for a short time in paediatric intensive care or look after sick children for short periods prior to retrieval to a paediatric intensive care unit. It is not intended to be a complete guide but rather a synopsis of the most salient points. With this in mind, we hope to have written it in an easily readable form.

The book is in three sections. The first is about basic principles of intensive care. The second section deals with specific conditions through different systems. The final section is a section on drugs which are commonly used in the critically ill child. We apologise for any omissions.

We would like to thank Dr Monica Stokes from Birmingham Children's Hospital for the chapter on Cardiac Problems on the PICU. We would also like to thank the editorial staff at GMM for their infinite patience and persistence. Finally we would like to thank Judy Needham for her secretarial assistance.

C G Stack
P Dobbs

October 2003

Section 1

Basic Principles of PICU

CHAPTER 1

DIFFERENCES BETWEEN THE CHILD, THE NEONATE AND THE ADULT

Children are not just small adults. Various anatomical, physiological and pharmacological differences occur. The differences are significant and there is a continuous and variable change from the neonate onwards. This chapter covers the relevant differences between neonates and adults.

Anatomy and physiology

Airway

Neonates have relative to adults:

- the cricoid ring which is the narrowest part of the airway in the child; the vocal cords are in the adult
- the cricoid cartilage which is a full ring of cartilage
- large tongue
- large omega shaped epiglottis
- anterior larynx which is at a higher level
- large head
- short trachea, greater angle of carina; left main bronchus more horizontal
- the nasal passage which is approximately the same size as the cricoid ring in children
- obligate nose breathers

Problems/relevance

- for basic airway management the head needs to be in the neutral position
- tend to be more difficult to intubate than older child or adult
- a straight bladed laryngoscope is needed to lift the epiglottis in children up to about 2 years of age to give a better view of the vocal cords
- uncuffed endotracheal tubes are used up to about 10 years of age to reduce the risk of sub-glottic oedema and long-term sub-glottic stenosis
- risk of endobronchial intubation (tubes too long)

Breathing

- alveoli increase mainly in number in infants and in size in older children
- bronchi have relatively more cartilage, less muscle and more glands
- small airway obstruction is more likely to be due to inflammation and oedema in infants and muscle spasm in older children

1

Table 1.1 Respiratory rates in children by age

Age	Rate (breaths/min)
<1	30–40
1–2	25–35
2–5	25–30
5–12	20–25
>12	15–20
Adult	12–15

- ribs more horizontal
- breathing is diaphragmatic
- greater elasticity of chest wall
- the diaphragm and intercostal muscles have fewer Type I muscle fibres which are adapted for sustained activity
- leads to relatively earlier tiring of these muscles
- faster respiratory rate 30–40 bpm at birth (Table 1.1)
- respiration often irregular with apnoeas particularly in premature infants
- similar tidal volume, compliance per kg compared to adults
- neonates have higher oxygen consumption, higher closing volumes and increased V/Q mismatch leading to lower PaO_2
- reduced oxygen reserve
- chemoreceptors have a more effective response to CO_2 rise than oxygen fall
- fall in oxygen tension stimulates respiration but only briefly in neonates
- surfactant production is reduced in premature babies, infant respiratory distress syndrome, bronchiolitis, adult respiratory distress syndrome (ARDS), pulmonary oedema and pneumonia
- more likely to have respiratory rather than cardiac arrest

Problems/relevance
Signs of increased work of breathing include:

- increased respiratory rate
- intercostal, subcostal recession due to the elastic chest wall
- use of accessory muscles, nasal flaring, grunting
- sweating and anxiety
- diaphragmatic splinting (e.g. air in stomach) may compromise respiration
- 50% of airway resistance is in the nasal passages
- tendency to have respiratory failure/arrest when critically ill

Table 1.2 Pulse rate and blood pressure by age

Age	Heart rate (bpm)	Systolic blood pressure (mmHg)
<1	110–160	70–90
1–2	100–150	80–95
2–5	95–140	80–100
5–12	80–120	90–110
>12	60–100	100–120

- in particular ex-premature neonates are prone to apnoeas
- bradycardia occurs often with hypoxia

Cardiovascular
- cardiac output is heart rate dependent in neonates
- stroke volume is fixed due to less compliant left ventricle
- relatively less intracellular calcium in neonates
- the myocardium is therefore more sensitive to parenterally administered calcium
- closure of foramen ovale and ductus arteriosus normally occurs during first 48 h of life with pulmonary vascular resistance and arterial pressure falling to normal by 2–4 weeks of age
- assessment in the child includes central capillary refill time (normal less than 2 s) or core-peripheral temperature difference (less than 2°C). Beware cold peripheries leading to a longer capillary refill time.
- palpation of the fontanelle can assist in assessment of fluid status in infants
- systolic blood pressure can be estimated by the formula:

$$80 + (\text{age in years} \times 2) \ (\text{Table 1.2})$$

Problems/relevance
- hypotension is a pre-terminal sign
- response to fluid loss is tachycardia and vasoconstriction, leading to increased capillary refill time and sometimes mottling and air hunger
- transitional circulation can persist precipitated by cold, hypoxia or acidosis. This leads to worsening hypoxia. Treatment is by hyperventilation with 100% oxygen, correction of precipitating factors, inotropes or vasodilators may be required.

CNS
- relatively larger brain in newborn and infants
- larger proportion of cardiac output goes to the brain
- myelination increases during first 2 years of life

1

- low myelin sheath thickness leads to slower nerve conduction
- blood-brain barrier is less well formed

Problems/relevance
- greater passage of some drugs especially opiates and barbiturates across blood-brain barrier
- more sensitive to sedative and analgesic drugs

Neuro-muscular junction
- formation of motor end plates is not complete at birth
- takes longer to recover after stimulation than in adults
- in the first few days of life, the immature neuro-muscular junction leads to greater sensitivity to non-depolarising muscle relaxants and relative resistance to depolarising relaxants (suxamethonium)

Renal
- immature at birth. Rapid improvement occurs after birth but the kidney is less efficient in premature infants.
- the proportion of cardiac output to the kidneys increases from 4–6% at birth to 20–25% when mature
- more flow to medulla and juxta-medullary apparatus than cortex in the newborn
- leads to difficulty in excreting sodium
- the low blood flow is the cause of low glomerular filtration rate (about one third that of adults) and therefore reduced excretion of some drugs
- difficult to cope with water load
- unable to concentrate urine as efficiently
- ability to excrete acid reduced in first week of life

Temperature control
- skin fully developed by 32 weeks gestation
- greater surface area to volume ratio than in adults
- head has a greater surface area leading to heat loss
- also fluid losses greater in premature infants compared to term infants. In addition the greater surface area to weight ratio of infants over children leads to greater fluid loss.
- main heat production is by non-shivering thermogenesis by increasing brown fat metabolism in the first few hours of life. This leads to increased oxygen consumption.
- sweat glands more inefficient and therefore easier for the infant to become hyperthermic
- in colder environmental temperatures, heat loss occurs by radiation, conduction and convection

- prematurity increases heat losses for the same environmental temperature compared to term infant

Problems/relevance
- quickly cool down if left exposed
- need to keep warm either by wrapping or heating devices
- increased fluid requirements in neonates relative to older children

Blood
- blood volume is increased in neonates (90 ml/kg)
- haemoglobin F (HbF) predominant at birth. Only small amounts remain by 6 months of age.
- HbF has a greater affinity for oxygen than haemoglobin A
- oxygen dissociation curve is shifted to the left
- therefore oxygen is less readily given up to tissues
- physiological anaemia is maximal at 3 months and tends to be lower the smaller the infant at birth

Pharmacology
Pharmacokinetics is the quantitative assessment of absorption, distribution, metabolism and excretion of a drug. Also described as how the body deals with a drug.

Pharmacodynamics is the biochemical and physiological effects of drugs or what the drug does to the body.

- To produce a predictable and safe pharmacological response it is important to understand the physiological differences that occur as neonates evolve to children and then adults.
- In general for many drugs, there is a period of sensitivity in neonates followed by a relative resistance in infants and young children and then tending towards adult doses in adolescence.
- Remember that ill children are likely to be generally more sensitive to most drugs.

Pharmacokinetics
Absorption
- The intravenous route avoids problems with variability in drug absorption.
- Inhalation: The combination of a higher alveolar ventilation and relatively large cardiac output of the neonate causes a quicker equilibration of alveolar to tissue concentration of drug than in adulthood.
- Oral/nasogastric routes: The rate-limiting step for absorption for the upper gastrointestinal tract is the speed of gastric emptying. This is altered in patients who are ill, have suffered trauma or received drugs

that reduce gastric mobility such as morphine. The acidity of the stomach is lower in the newborn infant (higher pH).

- Rectal routes: The rectal route can be useful. Absorption can vary with pH (normal 7–12).
- Intramuscular: Children have a lower muscle mass as compared with adults but a higher cardiac output which ensures a reliable and rapid onset of action of intramuscular drugs. In conditions with a reduced cardiac output, onset may be delayed. The intramuscular route should be avoided as much as possible due to the dislike of painful injections.

Distribution
- When a drug is absorbed it will be distributed according to blood flow and the drug's solubility in that tissue.
- Neonates differ considerably from adults in that as the cardiac output is double that of adults, the circulating volume is relatively less leading to a much more rapid circulation time.
- The relative volumes of body compartments are also very different. The extracellular space in a neonate is 45% of body weight compared with only 20% in adults. Total body water is 80% in the neonate dropping to 55% in the adult.
- It would be expected that neonates would need a larger loading dose but due to the increased sensitivity at receptor level this is not the case.

Protein binding
- Infants have lower levels of proteins such as albumin, and binding sites are occupied by endogenous substances such as bilirubin. Drugs with a high affinity for albumin may displace bilirubin.
- Basic drugs such as opioids and local anaesthetics are bound to α_1-glycoprotein which only reaches adult levels at about 6 months of age. Hence in early life these drugs will have a much more potent effect due to the higher free fraction in the plasma.

Elimination
- Most drugs are metabolised by the liver to a more water soluble form and excreted by the kidneys.
- The liver is relatively large at birth, thus Phase I reactions in the liver (oxidation, hydrolysis and reduction) are relatively mature early on in life while Phase II reactions (mainly conjugation) develop more slowly.
- The kidney is immature at birth and takes up to 2 years to develop fully and this may delay excretion. Glomerular filtration rate is about one third that of adults at birth. Secretion and absorption within the tubule is less leading to reduced elimination of drugs such as penicillin and gentamicin.

Pharmacodynamics

Receptors: The differential maturity and numbers of receptors may explain some of the differences in dose requirements in neonates. For example neonates are particularly sensitive to non-depolarising neuro-muscular agents and resistant to depolarising neuro-muscular agents.

DIFFERENCES BETWEEN THE CHILD, THE NEONATE AND THE ADULT

1

CHAPTER 2

NEONATAL PROBLEMS IN THE PICU

Although the majority of neonates or small infants are cared for on a neonatal intensive care unit (NICU) there are a substantial number which are cared for on a PICU. These will include those undergoing cardiac or general surgery (see separate chapters) and medical patients following discharge from the NICU. In particular, development of respiratory disorders (e.g. bronchiolitis) are common. The aim of this chapter is to consider some of the particular problems of neonates which may be encountered on the PICU.

Respiration
- foetal lung fluid production reduces during delivery
- the first breath generates a negative pressure in the lungs of up to 40 cm H_2O allowing air into the alveoli
- primary apnoea may occur due to asphyxia, prematurity, sepsis, trauma, congenital malformations or depressant drugs
- if respiration does not commence gasping occurs followed by terminal apnoea
- appropriate resuscitation should reverse this situation
- use APGAR scoring at 1 and 5 min to assess (see Table 2.1)
- respiratory compliance rapidly improves in the first hour of life

Respiratory distress syndrome
- follows surfactant deficiency in premature neonates
- symptoms are: tachypnoea, increased work of breathing, increased oxygen requirements within 4 h of birth
- leads to reticulo-granular appearance on X-ray
- injury because of infection or ventilation may lead to pulmonary interstitial emphysema (PIE) and later to chronic disease: broncho-pulmonary dysplasia (BPD)

Table 2.1 APGAR score is calculated at 1 and 5 min after delivery

Clinical feature	0	1	2
Heart rate	<60	60–100	>100
Respiration	Absent	Gasping or irregular	Regular
Muscle tone	Limp	Diminished or normal	Normal with active movements
Response to stimulation	Nil	Grimace	Cry
Colour	White	Blue	Pink

- early use of surfactant, nasal continuous positive airway pressure (CPAP) and high frequency oscillation has improved outcome
- complications include pneumothorax, pulmonary haemorrhage and pulmonary hypertension

Cardiovascular

Patent ductus arteriosus
- the ductus arteriosus usually closes within the first few days of life in response to a raised PaO_2
- it may remain patent (PDA) due to prematurity, illness or hypoxia
- closure may lead to the unmasking of congenital cardiac disease (see Chapter 12)
- symptoms include tachypnoea, pulmonary oedema and a continuous variable murmur heard posteriorly
- diagnosis by echocardiography
- treatment: medical by indomethacin, surgical via thoracotomy

Persistent foetal circulation
- the first breath expands the lungs, reducing the pulmonary vascular resistance and increasing the oxygen content of the blood
- pulmonary blood flow increases leading to an increase in left atrial pressure and closure of the foramen ovale
- cessation of flow to the placenta via the umbilical arteries leads to an increase in the systemic vascular resistance
- raised oxygen tension helps reduce pulmonary vascular resistance and should promote closure of the ductus arteriosus
- however, some conditions can lead to persistent foetal circulation or pulmonary hypertension of the newborn
- hypoxia, cold, pulmonary hypoplasia (congenital diaphragmatic hernia) predispose
- can also occur following the early post-operative period in neonatal cardiac surgery
- treatment includes hyperventilation with 100% oxygen, use of inhaled nitric oxide, treatment of the cause

Environment
- premature neonates lose heat rapidly and need to be kept in a thermo-neutral environment
- tend to be unable to respond to other stresses and become ill more quickly
- in general premature neonates do not respond well to handling and this should be kept to a minimum

Gastrointestinal
- physiological jaundice occurs normally after birth:
  - appears after 48 h

  - peaks by 5 days
  - returns to normal by 10 days (14 in the premature neonate)
  - unconjugated bilirubin
- can be abnormal – occurs too early, rises too fast, persists too long (Table 2.2)
- investigation includes blood cultures, virology, liver function tests (LFT's), Coombs test and appropriate tests if an inborn error of metabolism is suspected
- treatment of conjugated bilirubinaemia is dependent on age and bilirubin level
- phototherapy splits unconjugated bilirubin allowing excretion in urine and bile
- if the level is higher exchange transfusion may be required

Necrotising enterocolitis
- predominately premature infants, 3–10 days post-natal
- mortality 30–40%
- cause not definitely known but usually occurs in enterally fed babies and there are occasional epidemics
- early signs include abdominal distension, vomiting, bloody stools, apnoea or shock

Table 2.2 Causes of hyperbilirubinaemia in neonates

Type	Effect	Cause	Specific
Unconjugated	Intra-vascular haemolysis	Blood group incompatibility	Rhesus (Coombs +) ABO (Coombs –)
		Red cell fragility	Spherocytosis
		Inborn errors	G6PD, pyruvate kinase deficiency
	Polycythaemia	Twin to twin transfusion Placental transfusion Chronic hypoxia	
	Other red cell breakdown	Bruising from birth injury	Breech delivery, forceps
	Failure of conjugation	Inhibition	Breast milk
		Inborn error	Gilberts, Dubin-Johnson, Rotor, Crijer-Najer
	Other	Dehydration Sepsis	
Conjugated		Inborn errors	Galactosaemia, tyrosinaemia α_1-antitrypsin deficiency
	Obstruction	Biliary atresia	
	Infection	Hepatitis	

- may appear septic with disseminated intra-vascular coagulation (DIC), neutropaenia and thrombocytopaenia
- abdominal X-ray may reveal gas in the bowel wall or portal venous system; or free gas in the peritoneum
- treatment is supportive with IV fluids, inotropes, ventilation as necessary
- cessation of enteral feeding, TPN
- broad spectrum antibiotics
- review for bowel perforation
- surgical approach includes peritoneal drainage, or bowel resection often with defunctioning ileostomy

CNS

Intra-ventricular haemorrhage
- usually affects very small infants as a complication of severe illness including hypotension, hypoxia and acidosis
- diagnosis is by cranial ultrasound
- no treatment is available, therefore prevention is by avoiding precipitating causes including handling
- Table 2.3 describes the grades of intra-ventricular haemorrhage which can occur. Grades I and II usually are subsequently asymptomatic

Retinopathy of prematurity (retrolentral fibroplasia)
- disease of immature retina
- occurs because the normal growth of retinal vessels ceases and abnormal proliferation occurs into the vitreous humour. This can lead to retinal detachment and blindness.
- screen infants less than 30 weeks gestation or 1300 g birth weight
- also screen infants less than 35 weeks or 1800 g following supplemental oxygen
- consideration of this should be taken into account in the PICU, maintaining lower saturations in those babies than one would normally accept

Table 2.3 Grades of intra-ventricular haemorrhage

I	• arises from germinal matrix on floor of lateral ventricle but does not extend into the CSF
II	• extends into CSF without ventricular distension

III	• associated with ventricular distension
	• often symptomatic:
	  – systemic collapse with apnoea, acidosis, hypoxia, hypotension
	  – seizures

IV	• similar appearance to III with echogenicity in the peri-ventricular white matter • long-term hydrocephalus may arise • long-term outcome poor

2

CHAPTER 3

RESUSCITATION

A cardiac arrest occurs when there is an absence of a central pulse. In children a cardiac arrest is usually secondary to hypoxia or hypovolaemia. Rarely is it due to a structural defect except in neonates.

Management is divided into basic life support (Figure 3.1) and advanced life support.

- 'SAFE' approach
  Shout for help
  Approach with care
  Free from danger
  Evaluate ABC
- Stimulate and check responsiveness
  - Ask 'are you alright' – move child's arm, but take care if any suspected trauma to avoid cervical spine movement by holding head still

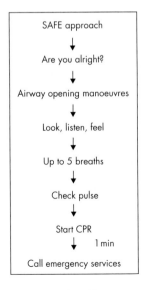

Figure 3.1 Basic life support

- Open airway with chin lift or jaw thrust (if suspected cervical injury)
- Check for breathing
  - Look for chest movement
  - Listen for breath sounds
  - Feel for exhaled breath
  - If breathing place the child in the recovery position
  - If not breathing give two effective breaths out of five attempts
- Check pulse for 10 s
  - brachial for infant
  - central (carotid or femoral) for child

If pulse >60 bpm within 10 s check for signs of breathing, if no breaths continue with rescue breathing.

- If inadequate circulation or no pulse commence chest compressions

Infant
- 1 fingerbreadth below inter-nipple line
- depress sternum using with two fingers by one third of depth of child's chest
- continue at a rate of 100 bpm
- cycle of 5 compressions to 1 breath

Small child <8 years
- lower half of sternum one fingerbreadth above xiphisternum depress sternum using the heel of one hand by approximately one third of depth of child's chest
- cycle of 5 compressions to 1 breath

Larger child >8 years
- lower half of sternum (2 fingerbreadths above xiphisternum)
- depress sternum using the heels of both hands with fingers interlocked
- sternum should be depressed by approximately one third of depth of child's chest
- 15 compressions to 2 breaths

In infants an alternative method for chest compressions when there is more than one rescuer is to encircle the child's chest with your hands and depress the sternum with both thumbs.

Continue resuscitation for 1 min and then go for help if alone, otherwise continue until help has arrived.

RESUSCITATION

3

Advanced life support

RESUSCITATION

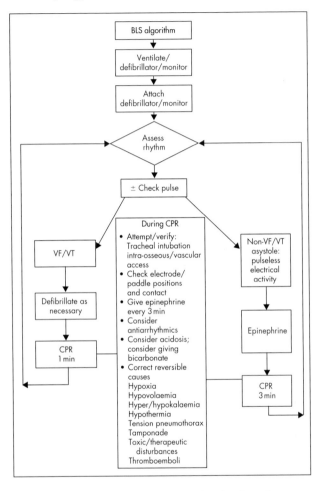

Figure 3.2 Paediatric advanced life support algorithm (from Resuscitation Council (UK) guidelines)

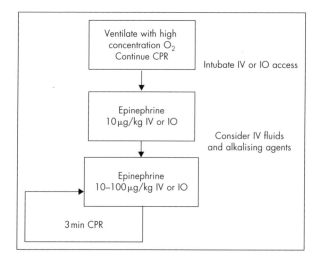

Figure 3.3 Protocol for asystole

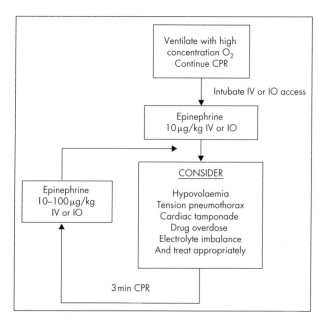

Figure 3.4 Protocol for pulseless electrical activity

RESUSCITATION

3

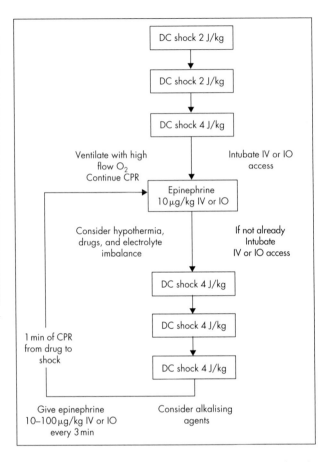

Figure 3.5 Protocol for ventricular fibrillation and pulseless ventricular tachycardia

Figures 3.2–3.5 give the algorithms for advanced life support and the commonest cardiac arrest scenarios in children: asystole, pulseless electrical activity and ventricular fibrillation.

Epinephrine (adrenaline)
Dose:

- venous or intra-osseous access: 10 μg/kg (0.1 ml/kg of 1:10 000 solution)
- no venous or intra-osseous access consider giving 100 μg/kg (1 ml/kg of 1:10 000 solution) via endotracheal tube

- higher doses (up to 100 μg/kg) may be given if there is intra-arterial blood pressure monitoring or if the arrest is secondary to extreme vasodilation, i.e. sepsis, anaphylaxis

Epinephrine is used to increase aortic diastolic pressure and thus improve coronary perfusion during cardio-pulmonary resuscitation (CPR).

Alkalising agents
Routine use of sodium bicarbonate has not been shown to be of benefit during cardiac arrests. It may be considered in prolonged arrests with severe metabolic acidosis and established ongoing ventilation. Dose 1 ml/kg of 8.4% solution.

Intra-venous fluids
20 ml/kg of crystalloid should be given if there is no response to the initial dose of epinephrine.

Anti-arrhythmic drugs
Amiodarone is the drug of choice in shock resistant VF and pulseless VT. Dose is 5 mg/kg IV as a bolus.

Allow 1 min for any drug to reach the heart.

RESUSCITATION

3

CHAPTER 4

THE STRUCTURED APPROACH TO THE SERIOUSLY INJURED CHILD

Trauma is the commonest cause of death in children over the age of one comprising approximately a quarter of all deaths in this age group. A trimodal distribution of deaths is described:

- within a few minutes due to injuries incompatible with life
- within a few hours due to respiratory or cardiovascular failure or raised intra-cranial pressure. These children will die without prompt intervention.
- within days due to multi-organ failure or infection which may be prevented by appropriate intensive care

The majority of deaths are associated with significant head injury.

When assessing and treating children, a system that ensures rapid assessment and identification of all problems with prompt resuscitation should be used. Effective communication and smooth transition of care to other professionals is necessary. A detailed secondary survey should be used. Life threatening injuries must be treated immediately when discovered.

Initial assessment – the primary survey
Airway
- Relieve airway obstruction – use jaw thrust rather than chin lift as this maintains the cervical spine in-line
- Check for foreign materials, e.g. food, vomit, blood, teeth under direct vision
- Stabilise the cervical spine to avoid the effects of spinal cord damage. Always assume there might be damage until proven otherwise.
- If intubation is required, rapid sequence induction should be used because of the risk of gastric aspiration. In-line stabilisation of the cervical spine by a second person should be undertaken. Oral intubation should be performed because the risks of nasal intubation include further damage, bleeding or potential infection if there is a base of skull fracture.
- Give 100% oxygen

Problems include:
- Injury to face and neck may complicate intubation due to bone fragments, haematoma, oedema
- Fractured larynx may occur with a neck injury. Loss of the airway on sedation and paralysis may occur.

Cervical spine

- This has to be considered at the same time as the airway. Once it is established that the airway is clear the cervical spine should be immobilised using a hard collar, sandbags and tape.
- Cervical cord injury is rare in children, but it may occur without radiological abnormality because of the flexibility of the cervical spine (Significant cervical injury without radiological abnormality – SCIWORA)
- Lateral X-ray of the cervical spine needs to be part of the primary assessment of the injury
- Injury may not be apparent even if a cervical collar is in place
- Pseudosubluxation of C2 on C3 and of C3 on C4 can occur in up to 10% of normal children
- Most injuries occur through ligaments or discs, most commonly at C1–3 due to the large head on relatively weak neck muscles or at C7/T1
- Cervical spine injury can only be adequately excluded by a normal clinical neurological examination and the absence of pain in the neck
- MRI of the cervical spine may help in patients who are unable to communicate
- Cervical spine stabilisation should be maintained during transport, log rolling and waking
- The hard collar does cause an increase in venous pressure which may compromise cerebral perfusion pressure and therefore can be removed if the head is kept in-line particularly if the patient is sedated and paralysed by neuro-muscular blocking drugs

Breathing

Once the airway is secure then assessment of breathing can occur

- look for the work of breathing
  - presence of recession
  - respiratory rate
  - respiratory noises
  - accessory muscle use
- look for the efficiency of breathing
  - equal breath sounds
  - tracheal deviation
  - open chest wounds
- look for the effects of inadequate breathing on other systems
  - reduced consciousness
  - poor circulation and skin colour
  - high/low heart rate

THE STRUCTURED APPROACH TO THE
SERIOUSLY INJURED CHILD

4

Table 4.1 Treatment of breathing

- 100% O_2 via mask with reservoir bag
- Bag and mask ventilation
- Intubation and ventilation

Table 4.2 The AVPU scale

A – Alert
V – Respond to voice
P – Respond to pain
U – Unresponsive

If there is a deficiency in the breathing assessment this should be addressed prior to assessing the circulation (Table 4.1).

Circulation
- Rapid assessment of circulation – heart rate, capillary refill time, pulse volume
- Consider also blood pressure, skin colour and temperature, respiratory rate and mental status
- Remember systolic blood pressure is maintained relatively late in the shocked state

Signs of significant blood loss are:
- tachycardia
- cool pale or mottled skin
- tachypnoea
- mental agitation

Signs of severe blood loss are:
- tachycardia/bradycardia
- falling BP
- sighing respiration
- reduced conscious level

Vital signs vary with age in children (see Chapter 1 for the normal values).

Treatment
- 2 large IV cannulae
- Bloods for FBC, U + E, X-match, glucose
- Fluid bolus 20 ml/kg, 0.9% NaCl
- Fluid bolus 20 ml/kg colloid or crystalloid
- Blood 20 ml/kg
- Remember to consider obvious sites of blood loss that can be rapidly controlled by a tourniquet, e.g. crushed foot
- Urgent surgery may be needed, e.g. for ruptured vessels

Disability
The initial assessment of mental disability is with the AVPU scale (Table 4.2). The scale is easy to repeat and consistent.

- Pupillary signs and posture also have to be assessed
- More definitive assessment of the neurological status requires use of the Glasgow Coma Scale (GCS) (see Chapter 14)
- P on the AVPU scale approximates to a GCS of 8 suggesting that intubation in order to protect the airway should be considered

Exposure
Full assessment of the child should occur but facilities to prevent the child becoming cold should be available. Avoid embarrassment.

X-rays
X-rays of the lateral cervical spine, chest and pelvis should be taken as part of the primary survey.

Detailed assessment – the secondary survey
- Following the initial assessment and resuscitation the clinician should ensure that a full history is obtained
- A detailed clinical examination from head to foot should be performed including log rolling and a management plan formed. This needs to include fundoscopy and any other X-rays required.
- Urinary catheter and nasogastric tube placement should be considered
- If the child deteriorates at any time then revert to the initial ABC survey and resuscitation measures as outlined above
- CT of the brain should be undertaken if required. This may require a general anaesthetic. At the same time consider an abdominal CT preferably double contrast to exclude injury to the abdominal contents.

Analgesia
Morphine 0.1 mg/kg IV should be considered for analgesia. This should be titrated against response and be dependent to some extent on the neurological status of the child.

Notes
- Need to be structured and thorough
- If the secondary survey is incomplete (e.g. by the need for urgent surgical intervention) this needs to be documented and handed over in order that it is completed when the patient is stabilised

THE STRUCTURED APPROACH TO THE SERIOUSLY INJURED CHILD

4

CHAPTER 5

AIRWAY AND VENTILATION

Maintenance of the airway is an essential core function in the critically ill child. Indications for intubation and the equipment and drugs needed are detailed in Tables 5.1 and 5.2.

Endotracheal tube requirements
- Internal diameter: (Age/4) + 4 mm (over 1 year old)
- Need half a size smaller and larger available when undertaking intubation

Table 5.1 Indications for intubation

Cardiac or respiratory arrest
Maintenance of airway
Patients requiring ventilation
- increasing oxygen requirements
- respiratory failure
- decreased level of consciousness
Potential airway obstruction, e.g. burn

Table 5.2 Requirements for intubation

Equipment	Drugs
Suction	Oxygen
Laryngoscopes (two working ones)	Anaesthetic/sedation agents
Oral airways	Muscle relaxant
Face masks	Atropine
Ventilation circuit	
Endotracheal tubes	
Magill's forceps	
Intubation aids, e.g. bougies	
Stethoscope	
Tape	
Carbon dioxide measurement	

Table 5.3 Endotracheal tubes for below 1 year of age

	internal diameter (mm)	oral length (cm)	nasal length (cm)
premature infant	2.5–3.0	5.5–7.0	7.0–9.0
newborn	3.0	8	10
6 months	3.5	10	12
1 year	3.5–4.0	11	14

- Length (Age/2) + 12 cm for oral
    (Age/2) + 15 cm for nasal
- Table 5.3 gives a guide to the size and length of endotracheal tubes in infants under 1 year of age
- As a rough estimate the same number of cm through the cords as the internal diameter in mm will lead to the endotracheal tube being in the correct place
- Remember to leave some extra for taping

Confirmation of successful intubation
- tube seen passing through vocal cords by direct vision
- confirmation that carbon dioxide is being expired
- auscultation may be misleading because sounds may be heard over the chest despite oesophageal intubation. Best to listen in both axillae and check over stomach.
- chest X-ray to check position – the tip should be around the level of the clavicles

Complications of intubation
- hypoxia
- failure
- misplacement (oesophageal intubation)
- trauma to lips, teeth, adenoids, soft tissues of oro or nasopharynx, larynx
- endobronchial intubation
- laryngospasm
- bradycardia/tachycardia
- sub-glottic oedema potentially leading to post-extubation stridor
- sub-glottic stenosis related to:
  - frequent reintubations
  - too tight an endotracheal tube
  - high pressure endotracheal tube cuffs

Criteria for extubation
- adequate oxygenation on FiO_2 <0.4
- adequate respiratory drive
- adequate recovery from neuro-muscular blockade and sedation
- intact cough and gag reflexes

Immediate complications of extubation
- Laryngospasm
- Pulmonary aspiration
- Bronchospasm
- Post-extubation stridor

Laryngospasm
- prevention by adequate patient arousal and suction of pharyngeal secretions
- treatment: 5–10 cm H_2O positive end expiratory pressure via bag and mask
- sedation, suxamethonium and reintubation if necessary

Post-extubation stridor
- may develop over first few minutes after extubation
- prevention:
  - leak around endotracheal tube prior to extubation
  - few reintubations
  - pre-extubation steroids: Dexamethasone for 24 h
- treatment:
  - nebulised adrenaline
    0.5 ml/kg 1:1000 to a maximum of 5 ml
    1:1000 3 hourly or 1 ml 1:1000 half hourly
  - steroids
  - reintubation usually with smaller diameter endotracheal tube

Oral endotracheal tubes
Advantages
- easy to insert
- rapid control of airway

Disadvantages
- patient discomfort – gagging
- obstruction by biting
- oral hygiene
- more difficult than nasal tubes to secure
- more movement in pharynx and larynx
- more sedation required and problems at extubation with oversedation when the stimulus of the tube is removed

Nasal endotracheal tubes
Advantages
- more comfortable, therefore less sedation required
- easier to fix
- less movement in nasopharynx and larynx
- can be used for a few weeks if necessary

Disadvantages
- more difficult to insert, using Magill's forceps, it may be necessary to direct the tube down the trachea

- nasal erosions
- false passage creation
- damage to nasopharynx on insertion
- potential risk of sinusitis
- more difficult to suction than an oral tube
- may kink at entrance of nostril or posteriorly in nasopharynx

Contra-indications
- bleeding diathesis
- basal skull fracture potentially leading to the development of meningitis
- anatomical problems such as choanal stenosis or facial deformities

Unlike adults, nasal tubes are preferred to oral tubes for children in most circumstances.

Tracheostomy
Advantages
- comfort
- less dead space
- easy suction for long-term use

Disadvantages
- surgical insertion in theatre required
- significant insertion complications, e.g. bleeding, false passage, hypoxia
- accidental removal may be life threatening
- other early complications include: subcutaneous emphysema, pneumothorax, thyroid injury
- sub-glottic stenosis more frequent the smaller the child
- other later complications: wound infection, tracheitis, aspiration, tracheal granulomas, secondary bleeding

Ventilation
- ventilation is a fundamental intervention in paediatric intensive care (Table 5.4)
- sometimes difficult to decide when to ventilate
  - hypoxia, e.g. PaO_2 <8 kPa on 60% oxygen
  - worsening hypercarbia or acidosis
  - deterioration in neurological status
- trends are better than absolute values
- when not to ventilate:
  - no likelihood of recovery
  - severe co-morbidity (ideally previously agreed with parents)

Table 5.4 Indications for ventilation

Cardiac or respiratory arrest
Apnoea
Accompanying protection of the airway
Respiratory disease, e.g. pneumonia, bronchiolitis, acute respiratory
  distress syndrome (ARDS)
Cardiovascular disease, e.g. shock, pulmonary oedema
CNS impairment, e.g. encephalopathy, coma, status epilepticus
Neuro-muscular disease, e.g. Guillain-Barre
Trauma – head injury, lung or chest wall injury
Post-operative, e.g. cardiac surgery, co-morbidity, neonatal
Facial/upper airway burns

Physiological effects of intermittent positive pressure ventilation (IPPV)

Respiratory
- may worsen V/Q mismatch by ventilating areas which are not perfused
- atelectasis occurs, reducing functional residual capacity (FRC) in the supine and anaesthetised child
- decreased pulmonary perfusion if cardiac output falls
- reduced surfactant production

Cardiovascular
- lung volume increases leading to:
  - increase in pulmonary vascular resistance
  - hyperinflation squeezes heart reducing cardiac output
  - release of factors causing reduced blood pressure
- raised intra-thoracic pressure:
  - reduces venous return due to increased right atrial pressure
  - direct effect on chambers of heart
  - reduces pressure gradient and therefore afterload for left ventricle

Positive effects
- improves alveolar expansion
- usually improves oxygenation
- allows easy removal of secretions
- allows adequate analgesia to be given to some patients, e.g. neonates, trauma

Goals of ventilation
The goal of ventilation is to maintain oxygenation. This is dependent on:
- inspired oxygen concentration
- mean airway pressure which is manipulated via tidal volume, positive end expiratory pressure (PEEP), I:E ratios

- re-expansion of atelectasis or collapsed lung segments, i.e. recruitment and keeping open of alveoli and the reduction of V/Q mismatch
- reduction in the work of breathing
- improve ventilation and avoid significant hypercapnia and acidosis
- avoid complications of ventilation

Aims of ventilation
- aim to ventilate for as short a time as possible
- ventilation is supportive not curative

Ventilation strategy
- depends on pathophysiology of illness
- aims to minimise lung damage
- lung damage depends on:
  - volutrauma
  - opening and closing of alveoli
- thus in general lower tidal volumes and application of PEEP reduce lung injury

Volume controlled ventilation
- developed from anaesthesia

Advantages
- maintains normo or hypocapnoea
- useful in conditions where this is important, e.g. raised intra-cranial pressure, head injury, encephalopathy, pulmonary hypertension

Disadvantages
- higher peak airway pressures
- potential of more barotrauma/volutrauma

Pressure controlled ventilation
Advantages
- reduction in barotrauma/volutrauma
- less dead space ventilation
- reduced mortality in ARDS in adults

Disadvantages
- permissive hypercapnoea
- respiratory acidosis
- may lead to increased intra-cranial pressure
- increased sedation requirements

Table 5.5 Indications for HFO

Infant respiratory distress syndrome (IRDS)
Premature neonates <1 kg
Air leak syndrome
Meconium aspiration
Diaphragmatic hernia
Persistent foetal circulation
ARDS
Recurrent pneumothorax

Other strategies
- 'best PEEP' optimise PEEP between 5 and 15 cm H_2O to improve oxygenation. Usually increasing PEEP does not compromise the venous return too seriously.
- prone ventilation
- reducing lung water by use of diuretics (aminophylline is synergistic in combination with frusemide)

High frequency oscillation (HFO) (Table 5.5)
- distending pressure (mean airway pressure) recruits alveoli and improves oxygenation
- increasing the inspiratory time may help increase oxygenation but may also lead to overdistension and air trapping
- oscillation at 3–15 Hz enables carbon dioxide elimination depending on amplitude of oscillation. Frequencies of 10–12 Hz are used in neonates, 8–10 Hz in infants, 5–10 Hz in children.
- depends on square of tidal volume and frequency: $Vt^2 \times f$
- therefore increasing the amplitude increases the tidal volume and decreases $PaCO_2$
- inspiration and expiration are active
- high lung volume strategy, commencing with mean airway pressure above that on previous conventional ventilation

Complications
- raised intra-thoracic pressure
- disconnection for suction
- mucus plugging can occur
- less tolerant of hypovolaemia or myocardial dysfunction
- may have rapid changes in PaO_2 and $PaCO_2$ on changing on and off conventional ventilation
- air leaks (pneumothorax, pneumomediastinum) can occur

Advantages
- less acute and chronic lung damage than those ventilated conventionally

- animal studies show less inflammatory response
- less volutrauma
- improves oxygenation in those children who are failing conventional ventilation
- reduces atelectasis
- early use has been shown to improve respiratory morbidity in neonates

Practical considerations
- the ventilator tubing is relatively non-compliant making the connection to the endotracheal tube more difficult (Sensormedics)
- conventional suction involves disconnection leading to loss of mean airway pressure and therefore alveolar recruitment
- commence with a mean airway pressure 2–6 cm H_2O above that on conventional ventilation and increase until oxygenation improves
- frequent chest X-rays (12 hourly for the first 24–48 h) are required to assess lung distension
- frequent arterial blood gases are required to assess CO_2 elimination

High frequency jet ventilation
- flow of gas jetted into proximal airway with/without conventional ventilation
- tracheal necrosis has been a complication
- seldom used

Surfactant
- deficiency in neonates leads to neonatal respiratory distress
- also deficient in ARDS and bronchiolitis
- use has had a major impact in neonatal intensive care in reducing the length of ventilation
- has been used in adult ARDS with no change in lung function or outcomes

Inhaled nitric oxide (iNO)
- nitric oxide is a potent vasodilator
- synthetised in body, acts on smooth muscle in the vasculature of circulation
- when inhaled, main effects are on pulmonary circulation thus should not cause systemic hypotension
- rapidly inactivated by binding to haemoglobin to form methaemoglobin

Uses
- decreases elevated pulmonary vascular resistance in patients with pulmonary hypertension – primary, secondary to cardiac/pulmonary disease or post-cardiac surgery

AIRWAY AND VENTILATION

5

- increases pulmonary blood flow through ventilated alveoli thus reducing ventilation-perfusion mismatch

Practical problems
- inhaled delivery
- rapid conversion to toxic higher oxides of nitrogen depending on oxygen concentration, length of time in contact and the square of the iNO concentration
- need careful monitoring of nitrogen dioxide to patient, scavenging and environmental monitoring
- electrochemical monitoring best
- maximum nitrogen dioxide levels should be 2 ppm
- not all patients are responders
- therefore if no response iNO should be weaned and stopped
- evidence of improvement in oxygenation but not definite evidence of improved survival
- high doses usually not more effective
- doses 0.1–1.0 ppm have been shown to have an effect although 10–20 ppm are often used
- discontinuation can lead to a rebound reduction in PaO_2 and therefore weaning can be difficult. This is possibly due to reduced endogenous production.
- some evidence that combining high frequency oscillation and iNO may be more effective
- one trial in adults demonstrated no difference in mortality but improved numbers alive and off ventilator at 28 days after 5 ppm iNO
- expensive

Side effects
- methaemoglobinaemia (especially in neonates because of combining with foetal haemoglobin). Treatment is with methylene blue 1 mg/kg.
- may cause systemic vasodilatation and may have a negative inotropic effect causing hypotension
- 50–60% nitrogen dioxide is retained in lung and reacts with water to form nitric and nitrous acids
- inhibits platelet aggregation
- nitrogen dioxide causes tachypnoea, respiratory difficulty leading to non-specific oedema and chemical pneumonitis

Liquid ventilation
- use of oxygen-carrying perfluoro-carbons
- reduce surface tension thus leading to recruited alveoli being kept open

- total liquid ventilation – tidal volume is essentially liquid. This needs dedicated ventilator and oxygenator.
- partial liquid ventilation – FRC filled with perfluoro-carbon. A conventional ventilator is used.
- some studies showing benefit in premature neonates

Extracorporeal membrane oxygenation (ECMO)
- external circuit allowing oxygenation and carbon dioxide removal
- there are two types:

Venoarterial:
- blood is taken from the right atrium and returned via the carotid artery
- permanent ligation of vessels used is often required
- bypasses pulmonary circulation allowing 'lung rest'
- can assist systemic circulation
- risk of arterial embolisation

Veno-venous:
- requires higher extracorporeal flows
- elevates mixed venous PO_2
- depends on patients' own cardiac output
- reduced risk of embolisation

Indications
- reversible lung pathology
- potential of good quality survival
- >2 kg
- ventilated less than 1 week

Clinical
- should be referred with an oxygenation index (OI) of 35–40

$$OI = \frac{FiO_2 \times mean\ airway\ pressure \times 100}{PaO_2\ (mmHg)\ (or\ kPa \times 7.5)}$$

- evidence of neonatal survival of 80%; paediatric around 50%
- used in meconium aspiration, persistent pulmonary hypertension of the newborn, respiratory distress syndrome, severe sepsis
- complications:
  - 24% have neurological abnormalities on ultrasound/CT
  - haemorrhage including intra-cranial haemorrhage
  - chronic lung disease
  - renal failure

AIRWAY AND VENTILATION

5

Weaning from ventilation

Background principles

- recovery from acute event
- stable cardiovascular system (may be on low dose inotropes however)
- normal electrolytes and haemoglobin concentration
- free from infection
- free from pain

Weaning criteria

- normal $PaCO_2$ (for that child)
- vital capacity 10–15 ml/kg
- tidal volume 4–5 ml/kg
- peak negative pressure >20 cm H_2O
- spontaneous minute ventilation <10 l/min
- PaO_2 >8 kPa on FiO_2 0.4
- pH >7.3

Methods

- To T piece – ideal after short term ventilation and rapid reduction of sedation, e.g. early post-operative period, head injury
- Synchronised intermittent mandatory ventilation:
  - reduce ventilator rate
  - in older children wean to continuous positive airway pressure (CPAP)
  - in neonates down to 5 bpm
  - reduce pressure support
  - reduce CPAP

Advantages of slow weaning include:

- allows slow recovery from sedation and analgesia
- enables the respiratory muscles to recommence activity with support
- allows patient to improve slowly

Problems with weaning

- disuse atrophy of respiratory muscles
- neurological weakness in PICU patient
- decrease ventilatory reserve, e.g. starvation
- ventilators may increase the work of breathing if not able to synchronise well with patient
- increased work of breathing due to poor compliance, e.g. bronchospasm, narrowed airway
- unrecognised illness, e.g. nosocomial pneumonia

- failure to clear secretions
- prolonged effects of sedative agents

Oxygen

One of the main aims of artificial ventilation is the prevention of hypoxia. Yet oxygen is a toxic drug which within a few minutes of breathing 100% leads to:

- painful tracheitis
- slightly reduced ventilation
- constriction of blood vessels
- reduced surfactant
- small reduction in heart rate and cardiac output
- depressed red blood cell formation with prolonged exposure
- atelectasis because of removal of nitrogen splinting

In neonates high oxygen may lead to retinopathy of prematurity:

- hyperoxia in neonates leading to proliferation of blood vessels within the retina
- aim to keep PaO_2 7–10 kPa; oxygen saturations 90–92%
- in general in children difficult to separate lung damage caused by high FiO_2 and mechanical ventilation per se

Effects of ventilation on the lung

- mechanical ventilation produces lung damage thought to be due to:
- volutrauma:
  - high-end inspiratory volume
  - repeated collapse and distension of alveoli and airways
  - in ARDS some lung units remain normal and these are likely to be damaged with high volume ventilation

Aim to:

- keep lung units open with PEEP
- avoid overdistension by limiting tidal volume and end expiratory pressure
- moderate permissive hypercapnoea
- need either to allow spontaneous respiration within the whole respiratory cycle or heavy sedation as it is uncomfortable to the patient or may lead the patient to fight the ventilator

Non-invasive ventilation

Various types of non-invasive ventilation are available.

- CPAP – face/nasal mask/nasal prong
  CPAP driver
- Bilevel positive airway pressure (BiPAP) – face/nasal mask

- External jacket ventilator providing constant pressure, oscillation or ventilation

Indications
- Avoidance of intubation
- Respiratory disease, e.g. bronchiolitis, tracheomalacia
- Neuro-muscular disease, e.g. muscular dystrophy
- Oncological/haematological failure where intubation and ventilation often leads to a high mortality rate, e.g. respiratory disease in a child with leukaemia during treatment with chemotherapy

Advantages
- Not intubated
- Avoids sedation
- Easily weaned
- Long-term survival in neuro-muscular disease is considerably improved

Disadvantages
- Difficult to give high oxygen concentrations
- Physiotherapy and suction more difficult
- May lead to gastric dilatation
- Cannot be used if severe cardiovascular or respiratory disease
- May not be tolerated
- Full face mask may be less safe if the patient vomits

CHAPTER 6

CIRCULATION AND RHYTHM DISTURBANCES

After assessment and immediate treatment of the airway and breathing, the circulation needs assessment (Table 6.1).

The acute emergency is dealt with in the chapter on Resuscitation. The aim of this chapter is to follow up these problems.

Shock (Table 6.2)
Shock has three phases (Table 6.3).

Table 6.1 Assessment of the cardiovascular system

- Pulse – rate, rhythm, fullness
- Capillary refill time or core-peripheral temperature difference
- Blood pressure
- Assessment of the effectiveness of circulation
  - Effect on other systems, e.g. conscious level, urine output
- ECG

Table 6.2 Causes of shock

Hypovolaemic
Distributive
Cardiogenic
Obstructive
Septic
Dissociative

Table 6.3 Phases of circulatory shock

Compensated
- The body compensates for the cause of shock by maintaining essential body functions: blood pressure, urine output, cardiac function, neurological status
- The commonest signs are tachycardia, normal or near normal blood pressure, reduced capillary refill time, cooling of the peripheries, reduced and concentrated urine

Uncompensated
- Circulatory compensation fails
- Fall in systolic blood pressure, acidosis, oliguria, reduced level of consciousness occurs
- Anaerobic metabolism increases leading to metabolic acidosis

Irreversible
- These processes become irreversible and death ensues

Shock is the clinical state of circulatory inadequacy when there is the disruption of tissue perfusion leading to inadequate supplies of oxygen and nutrients to and removal of metabolites from the cells of an end organ. This leads to distributed function of these organs.

Hypovolaemic shock

Causes

- Haemorrhage
- Fluid loss: diarrhoea and vomiting
  heat stroke
  diabetes insipidus
  gastrointestinal obstruction
- Redistribution: burns
  sepsis
  peritonitis

Care must be taken in trauma patients – as there can be considerable blood loss into the pleural or peritoneal cavities or from pelvic or lung bone fractures without obvious sites of bleeding.

Clinical presentation shows the effect of the body attempting to preserve fluid to maintain the intra-vascular volume.

- tachycardia
- decreased peripheral perfusion (increased capillary refill time)
- reduced urine output
- decreased cardiac output
- normal systolic blood pressure

Distributive shock

Causes

- Anaphylaxis to drugs, blood, latex, foods, insects
- Neurological injury – head injury, spinal shock
- Septic shock

Changes in the vasomotor tone may lead to shock by pooling of blood leading to hypotension. Neurogenic shock from brain stem injury or high spinal cord transection may also lead to hypotension, due to reduced sympathetic tone.

Cardiogenic

Failure of the heart pump:

- congenital cardiac repair
- cardiomyopathy
- myocarditis
- post-cardio-respiratory arrest

- arrhythmia induced
- trauma
- sepsis

Signs may include those of heart failure including tachycardia, raised jugular venous pressure, gallop rhythm, lung crepitations, enlarged liver.

Obstructive

This leads to obstruction of blood flow from the heart and shock. Causes include:

- Pulmonary embolism by thrombus, fat or air
- Cardiac lesions, e.g. aortic stenosis, coarctation or interrupted aortic arch
- Tension pneumothorax
- Cardiac tamponade

Septic shock

Infection can cause overwhelming shock either as the primary cause or after release of bacteria from the GI tract has features of hypo-volaemia, distributive and cardiogenic shock. The features show signs of infection and a generalised inflammatory response leading to multi-organ system failure (MOSF) (Table 6.4).

Meningococcal septicaemia (see Chapter 20) is the most florid example of this syndrome but it may occur with other infections.

Dissociative

Here the cause is essentially the failure of the circulatory system to transport oxygen. Causes include:

- anaemia
- methaemoglobinaemia
- carbon monoxide poisoning

Table 6.4 Signs and symptoms of septic shock

- Tachycardia
- Hyperdynamic circulation leading to poor peripheral perfusion
- Tachypnoea
- Oliguria
- Lactic acidosis
- Fever
- Reduced cerebral function
- Disseminated intravascular coagulation (DIC)
- Hypoxaemia
- Renal failure

CIRCULATION AND RHYTHM DISTURBANCES

6

Inotropic and vasoactive substances

Inotropes and other vasoactive substances are used to support the heart and circulation in times of inadequate or inappropriately distributed perfusion, i.e. shock.

- In any patient there may be multiple forms of shock occurring at any one time.
- Before starting any vasoactive substance, intra-vascular oxygenation and fluid status should be assessed and corrected.
- If more than 40 ml/kg of fluid, crystalloid or colloid is required then inotropes should be considered.

General comments on inotropes

- Correction of acidosis and low phosphate help the inotropic effects of these agents
- Need to be given by central venous access except for low concentration dobutamine
- Inotropes increase urine output by increasing cardiac output
- Dose requirement will vary and often more is required than the recommended doses as there is a large interpatient variation between infused dose and plasma concentration
- Important to give appropriate fluid to maintain normovolaemia
- Combination of inotropes may be useful, e.g. dobutamine and noradrenaline
- With time there is receptor desensitisation leading to tachyphylaxis. Steroids may reverse this process.

Mechanism of action

Most vasoactive drugs interact with adrenergic receptors with variable selectivity to produce inotropy, chronotropy or vasoconstriction (see Table 6.5). Other drugs cause inotropy by increasing cyclic AMP (milrinone) or intra-cellular calcium (digoxin).

Table 6.5 Effect of inotropes on catecholamine receptors

	$\alpha 1$	$\alpha 2$	$\beta 1$	$\beta 2$	DA1	DA2
Epinephrine						
low dose	+	0	+	+	NA	NA
medium dose	++	+	++	+	NA	NA
high dose	+++	+++	+++	++	NA	NA
Norepinephrine	+++	+++	++	0	NA	NA
Dopamine	+−+++	+	+−+++	0−+++	++	+
Dopexamine	0	0	+	++	+	+
Dobutamine	+	0	++	+	NA	NA

Catecholamines

The catecholamine receptors have the following cardiovascular effects:

- $\alpha 1$ vasoconstriction
- $\alpha 2$ vasoconstriction
- $\beta 1$ increased contractility, increased chronotropy
- $\beta 2$ relaxation at smooth muscle – lungs, vessels – vasodilation, increased contractility
- DA1 renal vasodilation and natresis
- DA2 renal vasodilation and natresis

Formulae for drug delivery

Epinephrine/norepinephrine:

$$0.3 \times wt(kg) \text{ in } 50\,ml \text{ is equivalent to } 1\,ml/h = 0.1\,\mu g/kg/min$$

Dobutamine/dopamine:

$$30 \times wt(kg) \text{ in } 50\,ml \text{ is equivalent to } 1\,ml/h = 10\,\mu g/kg/min$$

Peripheral dobutamine:

$$3 \times wt(kg) \text{ in } 50\,ml \text{ is equivalent to } 1\,ml/h = 1\,\mu g/kg/min$$

The choice of drug depends on the patients' current cardiovascular state. Invasive monitoring will be required to assess BP and filling pressures.

- Dobutamine is a good initial inotrope which can be given peripherally. It causes positive inotropy and chronotropy and some vasodilation. In general it improves cardiac output rather than blood pressure.
- In a high output state (e.g. sepsis) norepinephrine may improve organ perfusion by increasing afterload.
- Epinephrine is used for positive inotropy with some vasoconstriction.
- Both dobutamine and dopamine act partially by adrenaline release from neurones.
- In a failing heart (e.g. cardiomyopathy) inotropy with reduced afterload may be required – dobutamine, dopexamine or milrinone may all improve the cardiac status.
- Dopamine was thought to increase renal perfusion at low dose and provide both inotropy and vasoconstriction depending on the infused dose. However the effects are not predictable and dopamine may have detrimental effects on the immune system and worsen renal failure in higher doses.

6

Phosphodiesterase inhibitors
- Inhibit cycle AMP breakdown in the cell
- Aminophylline is a strong chronotrope, vasodilator and weak diuretic
- Enoximone and milrinone cause vasodilation and increase in cardiac output
- Use in shock with high systemic vascular resistance
- May be useful in heart failure
- More effective combined with β1 stimulation from catecholamines than alone
- Increase cardiac output without increasing myocardial oxygen consumption

Other agents with inotropic effects
Digoxin
- Inhibits the sodium pump (Na^+/K^+ ATPase) leading to an increase in intra-cellular calcium
- Has negative chronotropic effects by increasing the refractory period of the action potential and also it reduces the conduction velocity of the AV node
- May be of use in atrial fibrillation

Calcium
- May be reduced post-bypass, in sepsis and following blood transfusions, possibly due to the citrate in blood products
- Infusions have vasoconstrictive and inotropic actions
- More effective in neonates than as the age of the patient rises
- Should be used if refractory hypotension with low ionised calcium
- Evidence that it may worsen the situation in sick cells

Triiodothyronine (T3)
- Essential for maturation of calcium channels in the sarcolemma and calcium ATPase in cells
- Reduced after cardio-pulmonary bypass, in sepsis and hypothermia
- T3 therapy reduced inotrope requirement in adults and improves myocardial function after cardiac surgery in infants and children
- T3 has effects on protein synthesis (slow) and effects on calcium ATPase activity to enhance diastolic relaxation of cardiac muscle and contractility
- Effectively acts as positive inotrope and vasodilator

CHAPTER 7

SEDATION AND ANALGESIA IN PICU

Sedation and analgesia are important for a variety of reasons within the PICU:

- to reduce distress
- to reduce the stress of critical illness (improve outcome)
- to reduce discomfort and pain
- to protect the child from injury and to allow medical care to be given
- to reduce parental stress of seeing their child distressed

Assessment

Many ways have been developed for scoring pain with faces, various colours, ladders, etc., but these rely on subjective assessment and sufficient watchfulness to be useful. Various scoring systems have been developed for assessing sedation of ventilated children. An example is the COMFORT score which looks at physiological variables:

- alertness
- heart rate
- respiratory response
- mean arterial blood pressure
- calmness/agitation
- physical movement
- muscle tone
- facial tension

There is some evidence that bispectral analysis may be useful in determining level of sedation and anaesthesia.

The assessment of adequacy of pain relief and sedation can be difficult. A number of factors need to be considered:

- nature of discomfort (e.g. ventilation)
- variations in physiological parameters (HR, BP, sweating)
- facial expressions/postures
- parental concerns

Management

There are several approaches to treating the anxiety and discomfort that may be experienced in ICU.

- psychological aids such as pre-warning/visiting PICU, explanations of what it is like
- parental presence and reassurance may reduce pharmacological requirements

- avoidance of psychological factors that may cause distress such as thirst and hunger
- regional nerve blocks to reduce pain and help to minimise the discomfort that can occur

A recent review of selective practice in the UK showed that the majority of paediatric intensive care units use a combination of opiate and benzodiazepine by infusion for sedation of critically ill children.

Complications
- Oversedation leading to coma, bradycardia, hypotension, respiratory depression
- Ileus
- Contribution to critical illness neuropathy
- Undersedation leading to pain, fear, anxiety, fighting the ventilator, accidental extubation

Anaesthesia
Induction of anaesthesia for intubation of the critically ill child can be fraught with problems. Most anaesthetic agents can cause hypotension particularly in hypovolaemic patients. There are two main techniques for induction: inhalational or intra-venous.

Inhalational anaesthesia
- This is used for patients with airway compromise where potential loss of the airway with neuro-muscular blockade or respiratory depression may lead to hypoxia
- Patients with epiglottitis, croup or other upper airway compromise should receive an inhalational induction
- Advantages include maintenance of the airway reflexes for a longer duration
- Care must be taken as children with partially obstructed airways take longer to become anaesthetised than normal children
- Disadvantages include the need for experienced personnel, may not be tolerated by the patient and hypotension through vasodilation and myocardial depression

Intra-venous induction
- This allows rapid and smooth induction in the emergency patient with early control of the airway
- Disadvantages include loss of airway reflexes, apnoea, hypotension due to vasodilation and myocardial depression
- Rapid sequence induction (RSI) needs to be performed if the child has risk of a full stomach. It has the advantage of rapid airway control.
- RSI needs a skilled assistant to perform cricoid pressure until the endotracheal tube is safely inserted

Table 7.1 Intra-venous induction agents

Drug	Dose	Side effects examples
Thiopentone (25 mg/ml)	3–5 mg/kg	Hypotension, myocardial depression Accumulates with more than one dose Pain if extravasates Intra-arterial injection causes thrombosis Histamine release
Propofol (10 mg/ml)	2–4 mg/kg	Has caused epileptic effects Hypotension due to vasodilation Pain on injection (mix with lignocaine) Often have movements after induction Avoid infusions
Etomidate (2 mg/ml)	0.3 mg/kg	Cardiovascularly stable Abnormal movements after induction Pain on injection Seldom used
Ketamine (10 or 50 mg/ml)	1–2 mg/kg or IM 10 mg/kg	Causes dissociative anaesthesia for about 20 min Cardiovascularly stable Provides analgesia Does not depress respiratory or cardiovascular systems Increases intra-cranial pressure Causes hallucinations

SEDATION AND ANALGESIA IN PICU

- Preoxygenation for at least 3 min with 100% oxygen via a close fitting face mask needs to be undertaken
- Anaesthetic induction agent, e.g. thiopentone (see Table 7.1) is given followed by suxamethonium to facilitate rapid intubation
- Laryngoscopy and intubation is stressful and often tachycardia and hypertension may ensue. The use of a short acting opiate in addition such as alfentanil may ablate some of this response.
- The use of a straight bladed laryngoscope may cause stimulation of the vagal nerve from the back of the epiglottis leading to bradycardia. Suxamethonium can also cause bradycardia either with the second dose or with the first dose in neonates and young infants. Atropine should always be readily available.

Sedatives and opiates
- midazolam is the commonest benzodiazepine used in paediatric intensive care
- no analgesic effects
- sedative, anxiolytic, amnesic, anti-convulsant
- breakdown products have activity, e.g. midazolam (diazepam) lasts for 10–20 h

7

- midazolam has a very variable elimination half life in critically ill patients especially in neonates
- hepatic dysfunction may prolong action
- lorazepam slower onset and longer action and has no active metabolite
- side effects include a withdrawal syndrome with hallucinations and jitteriness. This occurs especially after high doses of more than 1–2 weeks duration.
- can use 'drug holidays' by rotating the drugs used
- reduction of benzodiazepine slowly with substitution of other drugs orally (e.g. chloral hydrate or clonidine) can help reduce withdrawal
- propofol has been implicated in a number of deaths in children following 3 or more days of use usually in patients with pyrexia from an upper respiratory tract infection. The recommendation is not to use it below the age of 16, although it was useful in patients who were to be ventilated for a short time after head injury.
- ketamine is fairly useful as an analgesic but needs to be given with benzodiazepines to prevent hallucinogenic side effects
- clonidine is another useful sedative either orally or by infusion. It is useful in morphine withdrawal but is limited by its need to be withdrawn slowly otherwise rebound hypertension can occur (Table 7.2 and 7.3).

Neuro-muscular blockade
Indications for neuro-muscular blockade include:

- intubation and procedures
- as an aid to ventilation if the patient is fighting the ventilator or shivering
- to help control raised intra-cranial pressure
- in general it is better not to have patients paralysed as they are able to breathe, to move to reduce potential oedema and to allow assessment of sedation and analgesia thus avoiding possible awareness while paralysed
- patients who are paralysed for prolonged periods are more likely to develop critical illness neuropathy
- there are no real advantages to any of the non-depolarising muscle relaxants except that atracurium degrades depending on pH and temperature. This can be a problem in a warm PICU as the drug is affected by the environmental temperature, but is an advantage in patients with hepatic or renal failure (Table 7.4).

Regional anaesthetic techniques
Epidurals
- Epidural analgesia involves the placement of an indwelling catheter into the epidural space in order to give local anaesthetic, usually bupivacaine or ropivacaine, with or without opiate to aid analgesia

Table 7.2 Sedatives used on PICU

Drug	Dose	Comments
Midazolam	2–6 µg/kg/min infusion	• Accumulates • Care in hepatic dysfunction and in neonates • Problems with withdrawal
Lorazepam	0.1 mg/kg IV bolus	• Long acting
Chloral hydrate	25–50 mg/kg oral or rectal	• Can accumulate • Can cause hypotension • May be prolonged in neonates • Minimal respiratory depression
Propofol	0.025–0.1 mg/kg/min IV infusion	• Short acting • Can cause hyperlipidaemia and has been implicated in some deaths. Not recommended for long-term infusion
Ketamine	0.5–2 mg/kg/h IV infusion	• Analgesic • Releases endogenous catecholamines • Contraindicated with elevated ICP • Need to administer benzodiazepine to avoid hallucinogenic side effects
Clonidine	0.4–1 µg/kg/h IV infusion or IV/po bolus up to 4 µg/kg/dose 6 hourly	• Anti-hypertensive, care with first dose and build up • Weaning must be slow otherwise rebound hypertension may occur • Useful in morphine withdrawal

Table 7.3 Opiates used on PICU

Drug	Dose	Comments
Morphine	10–80 µg/kg/h bolus 0.1–0.2 mg/kg	• long duration • half life increased in neonates • easier to cross blood-brain barrier in neonates
Fentanyl	1–3 µg/kg/h	• longer duration than alfentanil
Alfentanil	10–50 µg/kg/h	• short duration of action • good cardiovascular stability

following surgery. Other indications include for flail chest where the analgesia provided may prevent invasive ventilation.

- the catheter has a number of centimetre marks to detect its position
- lumbar, thoracic or caudal epidurals can be performed
- usually centralised to area requiring analgesia
- regular measurement of the sensory block bilaterally is required to ensure that the block has not spread too far

Table 7.4 Neuro-muscular agents used on PICU

Drug	Intubation dose (also hourly infusion rate)	Comments
Atracurium	0.6 mg/kg	• degrades depending on pH and temperature not dependent on renal or hepatic metabolism • histamine release • tachyphylaxis occurs
Vecuronium or	0.1 mg/kg	• few side effects
Rocuronium	0.5 mg/kg	
Pancuronium	0.1 mg/kg	• vagolytic causing tachycardia
Suxamethonium	1–2 mg/kg	• depolarising agent for intubation • can cause hyperkalaemia in burns or neuro-muscular disease • raises ICP • bradycardia particularly after 2nd dose

Table 7.5 Complications of epidural block

- Failure – in particular unilateral block. May need top up bolus or to pull the catheter back slightly as it may be to one side
- Hypotension due to sympathetic blockade. Fluids and ephedrine may be necessary
- Dural tap leading to post-dural headache which is classically positional (sitting up), occipital or nuchal in location. Treatment includes analgesics and fluids
- Respiratory depression due to epidural opiate. Naloxone IV will reverse the respiratory effects but not the spinal analgesia
- Horner's syndrome
- Total central neurological blockade where the anaesthetic is injected into the spinal fluid leading to unconsciousness and hypotension. Treatment is supportive
- Other rare complications such as abscess and haematoma can occur

- caudal epidural catheters may be used in neonates for analgesia. Often these are by bolus 8–12 hourly.
- side effect of opiates in epidural analgesia may include itching and urinary retention (Table 7.5)

Nerve blocks

Various nerve blocks may be effective following trauma. Femoral nerve blocks are especially useful following fractures of the femur. Infusion through a catheter adjacent to the nerve can give long-term analgesia.

Simple analgesics
- These can be used as adjuncts for patients with post-operative pain, e.g. paracetamol, diclofenac, ibuprofen
- Improved analgesia occurs with regular use
- Remember potential side effects of NSAIDs with asthma and renal failure
- IV propacetamol (30 mg/kg qds) is a good alternative for patients who are nil by mouth and rectum

SEDATION AND ANALGESIA IN PICU

CHAPTER 8

FLUID, ELECTROLYTES AND NUTRITION

Fluid is required for:

- replacement of insensible losses
- continuation of essential urine output
- extra fluid for a modest state of diuresis
- replace abnormal losses

Normal maintenance requirements for children are dependent on weight. Requirements for neonates in the first week of life need to be reduced as they cannot excrete the fluid so easily. Fluid requirements increase on a daily basis to 150 ml/kg/day by about day 5 (Table 8.1).

Assessment

- major causes of fluid loss include gastroenteritis and diabetic keto-acidosis
- dehydration can be assessed by clinical signs and serum urea and electrolytes in combination (Table 8.2)

Table 8.1 Daily fluid requirements

kg	ml/kg/h
<3	6
3–10	4
11–20	2
>20	1

Table 8.2 Symptoms and signs of dehydration

Sign/symptoms	Mild <5%	Moderate 5–10%	Severe >10%	Notes/caveats
Decreased urine output	+	+	+	Beware watery diarrhoea making nappies appear 'wet'
Dry mouth	±	+	+	Mouth breathers are always dry
Decreased skin turgor	−	±	+	Beware thin skin, use several sites
Tachypnoea	−	±	+	Metabolic acidosis and pyrexia worsen this
Tachycardia	−	±	+	Hypovolaemia, pyrexia and irritability cause this

Table 8.3 Causes of increased and decreased fluid requirements

Increased
  Raised temperature (fever)
  Raised ambient temperature
  Neonates
  Radiant heater/phototherapy
  Burns
Decreased
  Humidified gases
  Neuro-muscular paralysis
  Hypothermia
  Renal failure

Table 8.4 Daily electrolyte requirements (mmol/kg/day)

kg	Na	K
0–10	2–4	1.5–2.5
11–20	1–2	0.5–1.5
>20	0.5–1	0.2–0.7

- part of a spectrum leading to hypovolaemic shock dependent to a certain extent on the speed of fluid loss
- hypovolaemic shock needs to be assessed and treated separately
- most of the body is water. 1 kg approximates 1000 ml.
- maintenance – fluid volume and sodium requirements dependent on weight
- deficit:

  % dehydration × weight × 10 = ml fluid required

  this is extra-cellular fluid – effectively 0.9% sodium chloride
- replacement fluid should be given over 24 h
- care with hypernatraemia (see below)
- 5% dehydration can be treated with oral electrolyte solutions. Greater than 5% requires IV fluids.
- Temperature increase/decrease by 1°C increases/decreases fluid requirements by about 7% (Table 8.3).

Sodium
Normal plasma level is: 133–144 mmol/l. Daily requirements are given in Table 8.4.

Hypernatraemia (greater than 150 mmol/l)
Causes
- vomiting/diarrhoea
- excess water loss, e.g. diabetes insipidus, osmotic diuretics, burns

- high sodium intake
- iatrogenic fluid restriction (often combined with drugs containing sodium)
- near drowning (seawater)

Presentation
- lethargy, irritability, coma
- seizures
- may be incidental finding in critically ill children
- mortality up to 45% in acute hypernatraemia with brain damage likely in survivors

Treatment
- treat underlying cause
- slow rehydration using sodium containing fluid, e.g. 0.45% saline with dextrose (over at least 48 h). May need 0.9% saline.
- reduction of sodium level slowly 0.5–1 mmol/l/h
- this is important because of the possibility of cerebral oedema and worsening coma
- death or long-term cerebral damage may occur
- desmopressin (DDAVP) can be used in diabetes insipidus to reduce water loss

Hyponatraemia
Causes
- Inappropriate antidiuretic hormone (ADH) secretion – decreased water clearance
- Water overload, e.g. iatrogenic, nephrotic syndrome
- Excessive sodium loss (e.g. diuretics, renal tubular dysfunction, diarrhoea and vomiting)
- Fluid sequestration, e.g. sepsis, burns

Symptoms
- range from non-symptomatic through lethargy to coma
- nausea and vomiting
- seizures usually below 125 mmol/l

Signs and symptoms depend on degree of cerebral swelling.

Therapy
- prevention by routine fluid restriction
- fluid restriction as therapy
- if symptomatic, 3% NaCl to return plasma sodium to 125 mmol/l 6 ml/kg of 3% saline increases body sodium by about 5 mmol/l. This fluid is irritant.

- frusemide will increase free water loss
- care to check for hypovolaemia
- in acute hyponatraemia, correction can be reasonably fast up to 125 mmol/l and then more slowly

Potassium
Normal serum level is 3.5–5.5 mmol/l

- Potassium is an intra-cellular ion and therefore plasma levels do not reflect total body potassium
- Large intra-cellular buffer, therefore abnormal levels reflect considerable variation from normal levels except if significant cell wall breach has occurred

Hypokalaemia
- common causes: diarrhoea, alkalosis, diuretics, volume depletion, hyperaldosteronism, beta adrenergic agonists in asthma
- secondary hyperaldosteronism may lead to hypokalaemia due to sodium and water loss
- signs – ECG changes: T wave inversion, ST depression, predisposition to dysrhythmias, skeletal and smooth muscle excitability and weakness
- treatment: the cause, oral or IV replacement

Kidneys are good at preserving potassium.

Hyperkalaemia
- causes: renal failure, metabolic acidosis, adrenal insufficiency, cell lysis, high intake
- hyperkalaemia can be accompanied by hypovolaemia in sepsis

Signs and symptoms
- risk of arrhythmias particularly levels above 7.5 mmol/l – can proceed to cardiac arrest
- peaked T waves, decreased R waves, widened QRS complex
- muscle weakness

Treatment (see figure 8.1)
- care with hypoglycaemia
- calcium resonium may lead to constipation
- work by redistributing potassium into cells

Calcium
Normal level 2.1–2.56 mmol/l

Hypercalcaemia
- rare
- causes: childhood malignancy, hyperparathyroidism

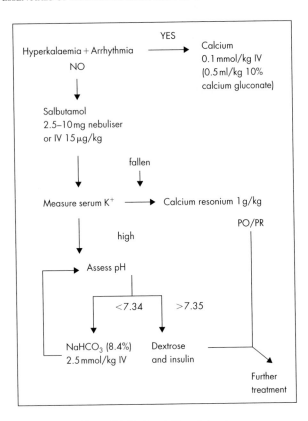

Figure 8.1 Treatment of hyperkalaemia

- iatrogenic administration
- effects: polyuria, kidney stone formation, hypertension, shortened QT interval and dysrhythmias
- treatment: hydration with or without diuretics, reduce calcium intake, phosphate infusion

Hypocalcaemia
- causes: severe septicaemia, rickets, hypoparathyroidism, pancreatitis rhabdomyolysis, citrate infusion (massive blood transfusion), acute and chronic renal failure
- treatment IV calcium
- may need infusion via central line
- high phosphate (especially in renal failure) may prevent rise

Magnesium
Normal level 0.64–1.09 mmol/l

Hypermagnesaemia
- very uncommon. Hypotension, coma, depressed reflexes.
- treatment: reduce intake, fluid, IV calcium

Hypomagnesaemia
- common up to 60–65% of adult ICU patients
- causes:
  - gastrointestinal: nasogastric losses, small bowel loss, malabsorption
  - renal: drugs including diuretics, intrinsic renal disease
  - post-transfusion
  - sepsis, burns

Effects
- ventricular dysrhythmias
- increase in PR and QT intervals, flat broad T waves on ECG
- neuro-muscular weakness
- may be associated with other electrolyte disturbances especially hypocalcaemia and hypokalaemia

Treatment
- IV bolus or infusion
- care with hypotension and dysrhythmias

Phosphate
Normal level 0.8–1.9 mmol/l

Hyperphosphataemia
Signs and symptoms:
- causes hypocalcaemia
- seizures and coma
- cause: excessive intake, reduced renal excretion due to reduced glomerular filtration rate, or increased renal threshold, cell lysis
- treatment: reduce intake, aluminium hydroxide antacids, restore plasma volume, insulin and glucose administration, dialysis, intra-venous calcium

Hypophosphataemia
- causes: reduced intake, increased loss, increased transfer into cells from extra-cellular fluid (ECF). Diabetic ketoacidosis and glycosuria, acidosis, renal tubular disorder, hypokalaemia.

- effects: reduced WBC phagocytosis,
    increased RBC production
    platelet destruction
    muscle weakness and peripheral neuropathy
    respiratory failure
    depressed myocardial function
    rhabdomyolysis
    CNS dysfunction/irritability up to seizures and coma
    liver failure
- treatment: prevention – TPN/enteral feed
    IV infusion except in hypercalcaemia, use low doses in hypocalcaemia
    risks include: hyperkalaemia, hypocalcaemia, hypomagnesaemia, hypotension, hyperosmolality, renal failure and calcium deposition

Acid-base disorders

- maintenance of a normal pH is essential for the functions of cells to be undertaken
- pH is normally within the range of 7.35–7.45. This corresponds to a hydrogen ion concentration of 35–45 nmol/l
- initially ill children often demonstrate abnormalities of acid-base homeostasis

Physiology
- Normal pH is maintained by buffers in the body. These are solutions which contain a weak acid and its conjugate base and are relatively resistant to changes in pH.
- Two main categories are bicarbonate and non-bicarbonate
- The non-bicarbonate forms almost 50% of the buffering capacity of whole blood. These are haemoglobin, plasma proteins and organic and inorganic phosphates.
- However, the bicarbonate buffer system along with plasma proteins are able to form the immediate response to an increase in acid or base
- The bicarbonate buffer system is dependent on the equation:

$$H^+ + HCO_3^- \rightleftharpoons H_2CO_3 \rightleftharpoons CO_2 + H_2O$$

- CO_2 (the acid component) is removed by the lungs and this mechanism can begin to act within minutes
- HCO_3^- (the base component) is regulated by the kidney, by the retention of HCO_3^- from the urine, greater production of HCO_3^- and increased H^+ excretion. This can act within hours.
- Full compensation by either mechanism is unusual

Table 8.5 Classifications, effects and causes of acid-base disorders

Respiratory acidosis
- Characterised by raised $PaCO_2$
- Hypoventilation due to
  - Respiratory depression
  - Obstructive and restrictive respiratory disease
  - Neuro-muscular weakness causing respiratory failure
  - Inadequate mechanical ventilation
- Increased CO_2 production
  - Seizures
  - Malignant hyperpyrexia
- Chronic respiratory acidosis is associated with a partially compensated picture with raised $PaCO_2$ and bicarbonate

Respiratory alkalosis
- Characterised by lowered $PaCO_2$
- Hyperventilation
  - Salicylate poisoning
  - Fever, sepsis
  - Encephalopathy
  - Hypoxic and acidotic patients may hyperventilate
  - Overventilated by mechanical ventilation

Metabolic acidosis
- Characterised by a rise in serum H^+
- Normal anion gap – HCO_3^- lost
  - From GI tract, e.g. diarrhoea, fistulae
  - From renal tract, e.g. proximal renal tubular acidosis, ureteral diversion surgery
- Increased anion gap acidosis
  - Renal failure
  - Ingestion, e.g. salicylates, methanol
  - Ketoacidosis, e.g. diabetic ketoacidosis
  - Lactic acidosis

Metabolic alkalosis
- Characterised by gain of HCO_3^- or loss of H^+
- Loss of H^+
  - Vomiting, e.g. pyloric stenosis
  - Gastric losses from nasogastric tube
  - Renal losses, e.g. diuretic therapy
  - Increased mineralocorticoids
  - Post-hypercapnia
- Increased HCO_3^- – administration
- Large citrate load, e.g. massive blood transfusion

- Acute rises in $[H^+]$ leads to an increase in intra-cellular cation leading to K^+ leaving the cell causing hyperkalaemia
- The anion gap can be used to estimate negative ions not measured regularly (Normal is around 12 mmol/l):

$$\text{anion gap} = \text{plasma } Na^+ - (\text{plasma } Cl + HCO_3^-)$$

- Table 8.5 and 8.6 give the classification of acid-base disorders and the signs of metabolic acidosis

FLUID, ELECTROLYTES AND NUTRITION

8

Table 8.6 Signs of metabolic acidosis

- Stimulation of respiration
- May become deep and sighing (Kussmaul's respiration)
- Myocardial depression, reduced cardiac output
- Peripheral vasodilatation leading to hypotension
- Confusion and drowsiness
- Reduced activity of inotropic agents

Table 8.7 Causes of lactic acidosis

Association with hypotension and/or severe tissue hypoxia
- Shock from any cause
- Respiratory failure
- Cyanide or carbon monoxide poisoning
- Severe anaemia

Associated with impaired mitochondrial respiration and increased lactate production
- Diabetes mellitus
- Hepatic failure
- Severe infection
- Drugs (e.g. salicylates)
- Toxins (e.g. ethanol)
- Inborn errors of metabolism

- Lactic acidosis is associated with an increase in pyruvate metabolism in muscle, skin and brain due to anaerobic respiration (Table 8.7).

Treatment

Respiratory acidosis
- Improve respiratory function by ventilatory support
- Need to be careful in patients with chronic respiratory acidosis

Respiratory alkalosis
- Treat cause in order to reduce respiratory rate and depth
- Reduction of ventilation or increase in dead space may help if ventilated

Metabolic acidosis
- Treatment of the cause
- Intra-venous fluids
- Sodium bicarbonate, but beware due to the left shift of the oxygen dissociation curve, inhibition of oxygen release from haemoglobin may occur
- Renal replacement therapy

Metabolic alkalosis
- Treat cause if possible (e.g. stop diuretics)

Table 8.8 Energy requirements

Age	kcal/kg/day
Premature neonate	150
Neonate	100–120
<10 kg	100
10–20 kg	1000 +50 kcal/kg over 10 kg
>20 kg	1000 +20 kcal/kg over 20 kg

- Saline responsive – those conditions with volume contraction of the extra-cellular fluid, e.g. via GI tract or kidneys
- Saline resistant (e.g. increased mineralocorticoid, hypercalcaemia) – treat the cause with adequate potassium and chloride replacement

Nutrition

Nutritional requirements (Table 8.8)

In critical illness nutrition may be poor due to:

- starvation due to illness and slow instigation of nutrition
- increased calorie use, e.g. from respiratory distress, pain
- effects of the critical illness: catabolism, pyrexia, stress

Poor nutrition may lead to:

- muscle atrophy and weakness
- decreased wound healing
- increased difficulty of weaning from ventilation
- reduced immune function
- atrophy of the gut mucosa

Assessment of malnutrition is difficult and no test (e.g. serum albumin) can easily diagnose this.

Aim is to help prevent the effects of poor nutrition particularly negative protein balance and try to maintain the immune response and wound healing.

Enteral nutrition

- try to instigate as early as possible if not contraindicated
- requires functioning gut
- preserves gut mucosa, possibly reducing chance of stress ulceration, even in small amounts
- cheaper and fewer complications than TPN
- bolus feeds more physiological
- may need to consider prokinetics or transpyloric tube to instigate successful feed

Complications
- Vomiting
- Aspiration
- Bacterial infection
- Blockage of nasogastric tubes
- Constipation – poor water intake
- Diarrhoea – may be due to infection, lack of fibre

Total parenteral nutrition
- commence early if enteral feeding failed
- requires central access if glucose is in high concentration
- increased septic complications
- metabolic and electrolyte imbalance particularly hyperglycaemia
- lipid, amino acids and triglycerides need checking at least weekly
- trace elements need checking if deficiency suspected
- long-term TPN may lead to liver failure probably due to cholestasis

CHAPTER 9

TRANSPORT OF THE CRITICALLY ILL CHILD

Sick children often need transportation within or between hospitals. Evidence from North America and Australia, shows that concentration of paediatric intensive care services into large units is beneficial and that outcomes, particularly in moderately ill children, are improved. Therefore to provide a more centralised service, transport of sick children is required between district general hospitals and the local paediatric intensive care unit. Patients transported by a non-specialised team into a paediatric intensive care unit compared to patients admitted directly to that unit demonstrated an excess morbidity due to intensive care related adverse events such as blocked endotracheal tubes. Physiological deterioration was similar in both groups.

Hazards of transfer

In one study 75% of children transferred between hospitals had one or more adverse events, which were of a critical or serious nature. Patients who subsequently died were more likely to have had critical events during transfer. If the escorting personnel were inexperienced there was more likely to be a critical incident. Reduction in morbidity has been shown by specialist teams. In one study, 4% of the patients suffered physiological deterioration during transfer by a specialised team. In the USA, a comparison of the transfer of sick children by specialised and non-specialised teams showed a significant reduction in intensive care related adverse events with the specialised team from 20% to 2%. However, when physiological adverse events were compared there was no significant difference between the two teams 11% for the specialised, 12% for the non-specialised.

Mode of transport

This depends on factors such as patient location, geography, distance and weather. The majority of transports are by local ambulance. Problems in the ambulance include lack of space and access, noise, light, temperature, the effects of motion including acceleration and braking and safety for staff and the patient. Air transport has the additional problems of extra noise, vibration, access, altitude and staff familiarity with the aircraft. The alteration in partial pressure of gases and gas filled cavities are potential problems. The use of pressurised aircraft is better. Fixed wing aircraft are easier to work within and have less noise and vibration than helicopters but are limited by the need to use a landing strip. It is only advantageous to use air transport if the trip by ambulance is longer than 2 h.

Staffing
Each patient transfer requires:
- an experienced specialist in Paediatric Intensive Care
- an experienced Paediatric Intensive Care Nurse
- trainee (medical and/or nursing)
  - the service should be consultant led. It should be available on a 24 h basis.

A paediatric intensive care nurse is an essential part of the team. They should be a senior staff nurse or above, to have reasonable experience on their own unit, be a registered IV giver and to have had experience as an observer on transfers prior to being a member of the team. There should be a sufficient pool of nurses able to be rostered as the retrieval nurse on a 24 h basis.

Equipment
Table 9.1 and 9.2 lists the essential equipment required for interhospital transfer. Appropriate sizes for all children need to be available.

Communication
- Discussion with the parents is required before transfer. This should include the reasons for transfer, treatment prior to departure and location of and visiting arrangements for the paediatric intensive care unit (Table 9.3).

Table 9.1 Essential equipment

- Monitoring
  - ECG, non-invasive and invasive blood pressure
  - oxygen saturation, end-tidal carbon dioxide
  - temperature
- Intubation equipment
  - masks and airways, endotracheal tubes
  - laryngoscopes, aids, e.g. Magill's forceps
- Cannulation
  - cannulae, CVP lines, intra-osseous needles
  - giving sets, syringes, needles
  - arterial giving sets
- Ventilator for both infants and children
- Manual ventilation circuits
- Suction
- Defibrillator (in ambulance)
- Stretcher – incubator
- Telephone, documentation, batteries, etc.

A comprehensive selection of drugs required because of:
- wide variety of potential illnesses of patients
- potential emergencies while in transit
- variable location of patient and therefore accessibility to drugs in referring hospital

---

Table 9.2 Essential drugs

Oxygen	
Cardiovascular	• resuscitation drugs
	• inotropes
Anaesthetic	• sedatives, relaxants
CNS	• anti-convulsants
	• antagonists, e.g. naloxone
	• mannitol
Antibiotics	
Miscellaneous	• steroids
	• diuretics
	• bronchodilators
	• local anaesthetic
	• saline, water, heparin
Fluids	• colloids, crystalloids

Table 9.3 Information required at initial contact by referring hospital

• Patient:	details, age, weight
• Illness:	diagnosis, identified problems, investigation results
	treatment undertaken
	appropriateness of referral
• Location:	hospital, ward, access
	medical staff contact, telephone number
• Advice:	bed availability PICU
	treatment
	your telephone number for further advice as required

• Contact should be at consultant to consultant level
• Responsibility including initial resuscitation and stabilisation remains that of the referring hospital until the arrival of the transport team. However all advice given by the PICU should be recorded.

• Transport of the parents, with their child, in the ambulance may be useful in the awake and anxious child but there are problems otherwise. This includes the lack of space, particularly if an emergency occurs; increased stress on both parents and staff and perhaps diversion of attention of the staff away from the child.

The ambulance journey
• The environment of the ambulance is hostile for the critically ill child
• It is small, cold, noisy and often has poor lighting
• Movement causes a number of problems. In particular, difficulty in monitoring of the patient, mechanical and by the staff, may lead to potential delays in recognition of critical events.
• Any procedures are very difficult to undertake while in transit
• There is the potential of motion sickness in the staff

9

Thus it is important to stabilise the child prior to transfer, protect the airway and have two working intra-venous lines. Consideration has to be given to restraint of the child on the stretcher or in the incubator in event of an accident or sudden braking. If, however, a problem occurs during transfer, it is safer to stop the ambulance and sort out the problem while stationary.

CHAPTER 10

DEATH ON THE PICU

The death of a child is often the saddest event of their life for a parent. It is against the natural law of survival which we have come to expect in the UK.

Mortality on PICU is about 5–10%. Many of these deaths may have been predictable at the time of admission such as a child with a severe head injury, or out of hospital cardio-respiratory arrest. Some may not, e.g. post-operative cardiac arrhythmia, meningococcal sepsis.

In all cases, the 'family' needs to be seen as the unit of care. Involvement of the family at all stages of their child's stay on PICU helps with the long-term outcome of bereavement. Regular communication with the medical staff and straightforward, consistent and unhurried explanations of what is happening to their child helps both parents. All the staff need to be aware of the different responses of the two sexes to their child's illness and death and the problems that this can cause within the family unit. Cultural and religious differences also vary leading to differences in response to death and the requirements for burial.

Withdrawal of intensive care

In 1997, the Royal College of Paediatrics and Child Health published a document discussing the withdrawal of treatment. Five situations were recognised:

- The brain dead child
- Permanent vegetative state
- The no chance situation – treatment delays death without alleviation of suffering
- The no purpose situation – the degree of physical or mental impairment is unreasonable for the child to bear it
- The unbearable situation where with progress and irreversible disease further treatment is more than can be done

Practical cessation of treatment

The end of life is hard even when expected. It is a difficult time for all concerned. Evidence shows that parents wish to be part of the decision and to be present even during resuscitation as this enables them to realise that everything was done for their child. Practical cessation of treatment includes:

- cardiac arrest
- brain stem death
- withdrawal of care with appropriate medication to prevent distress

DEATH ON THE PICU

10

Brain stem death

The Royal Colleges defined brain stem death as an indication that there is no longer any activity from the vital centres in the brain.

Two sets of tests of brain stem function are performed by doctors of more than 5 years post registration. The patient has officially died at the time of the first set of tests being negative. The second set are confirmatory only.

Prior to the tests certain criteria need to be fulfilled:

- a known cause for the coma
- the patient is normothermic
- normal biochemical and metabolic parameters
- no effects from sedation or neuro-muscular paralysis

The tests are:

- No pupil response to a bright light
- No corneal reflex
- No ocular response to caloric testing (ice cold water in the ear canal) (check that the ear drum is not perforated before testing)
- No gag reflex
- No cough reflex
- No evidence of cranial response to peripheral painful stimulus
- No respiratory effort to a raised carbon dioxide level (apnoea test)

Post mortem examination

There are certain circumstances in which a coroner's post mortem is essential, e.g. deaths associated with violence, post-operative within 24 h, accidents, poisoning. In other cases a hospital post mortem may help clarify the circumstances of death.

Following the Redfern Inquiry new consent forms for post mortem examination including information about retention of organs and tissue blocks have been introduced. Sensitivity with knowledge will help approach for permission. Cultural and religious differences exist towards post mortem examination. It is worth asking yourself if the examination would be useful.

Donation of organs for transplant

- Often raised by the family
- Permission should be sought sensitively
- Knowledge of the events and procedures following death can help allay doubts of the parents

Following death

- Be sensitive to religious practices
- Enable the family to have time with their child

- A follow up appointment about 6 weeks after death will help to answer questions and concerns of the family along with any results available from a post mortem

Information
- Resources for families and staff should be available
- A booklet allows relevant local information to be available
- A resource file will enable information to be available for staff

Section 2

Specific PICU Problems

CHAPTER 11

RESPIRATORY DISEASE

Respiratory

Respiratory illnesses that occur in children and necessitate intensive care can be divided into upper and lower respiratory obstruction and pneumonias. A further group may show inadequate respiration secondary to other diseases. These are discussed elsewhere.

Assessment of severity

Respiratory rate
- tachypnoea is the usual response to respiratory difficulty, but is also seen with metabolic acidosis and psychological disturbance (Table 11.1).

Increased work of respiration
- recession
  In younger children and infants the increased compliance of the chest wall makes recession a common sign. In older children (>7 years) it signifies severe respiratory problems. Both intercostal and sternal recession occur.
- use of accessory muscles
  Nasal flaring may indicate mild increase in work of breathing while sternomastoid, and other muscle use indicates markedly increased respiratory effort.
- grunting
  Grunting is due to decreased lower airway compliance. It is characteristically seen in infants and is a sign of severe respiratory difficulty. It may disappear in a fatigued child.

Effectiveness of breathing
The colour of a child's skin and mucus membranes give a subjective assessment of cyanosis. However the presence of anaemia, poor perfusion, hypercapnia or poor lighting complicate the assessment. Pulse oximetry should be used to give a more reproducible assessment.

Table 11.1 Normal respiratory rates

Age	Breaths/minute
<1	30–40
1–5	20–30
5–12	15–20
>12	12–16

Effect of respiration on other organs
Cardiovascular system – hypoxia initially causes a tachycardia which leads to bradycardia as it becomes more severe and pre-terminal.

CNS – hypoxia initially causes agitation then drowsiness and eventually coma.

Oxygen administration, and ventilation are the mainstay of treatment. These are discussed in Chapter 5.

Upper airway obstruction
Table 11.2 gives the causes of acute upper airway obstruction most of which are infective in cause. History of trauma or inhalation of a foreign body may differentiate the others. Table 11.3 gives a list of the main causes of congenital upper airway obstruction. These are more frequently seen by ENT colleagues but a child with a history of previous episodes of croup may have an underlying predisposition and need ENT referral when they have recovered from the acute illness.

Croup (laryngotracheobronchitis)
Croup is an acute viral upper respiratory tract infection. It is characterised by a group of symptoms – inspiratory stridor, barking cough, hoarseness and a degree of respiratory distress that increases with severity (Table 11.4 and 11.5).

Table 11.2 Acute causes of upper airway obstruction

Croup
Bacterial tracheitis
Epiglottitis
Diphtheria
Acute tonsillitis
Infectious mononucleosis
Retropharyngeal abscess
Trauma
Foreign body

Table 11.3 'Congenital' and non-acute causes of upper airway obstruction

Choanal atresia or stenosis
Laryngomalacia
Laryngeal webs, stenosis, cleft, cyst
Tracheomalacia (often associated with tracheo-oesphageal atresia)
Vascular ring
Bronchomalacia
Sub-glottic stenosis (acquired from previous intubations)
Laryngeal papillomata
Intra-thoracic tumours

11

Table 11.4 Clinical features of croup, bacterial tracheitis and epiglottitis

	Croup	Bacterial tracheitis	Epiglottitis
Commonest age	3 months–3 years	any age	2–7 years
Onset	gradual	gradual	rapid (hours)
Temperature	low or normal	usually high	high
Cough	barking/stridor	barking/stridor	muffled/none
Sore throat	no	no	yes
Posture	any	any	sitting forward
Drooling	no	no	yes
Voice	normal	normal	muffled
General appearance	non-toxic	toxic	toxic, anxious
Respiratory rate	rapid	normal	normal – early

Table 11.5 Common infective causes of croup

- Parainfluenzae virus
- Respiratory syncytial virus
- Adenovirus

Table 11.6 Clinical croup score

Parameter	0	1	2
Inspired breath sound	Normal	Harsh, rhonchi	Delayed
Stridor	None	Inspiratory	Inspiratory + expiratory
Cough	None	Hoarse cry	Bark
Retractions, flaring	None	Flaring and suprasternal retraction	Flaring, suprasternal + intercostal retraction
Cyanosis	None	In air	In 40% O_2

mild – score <2; moderate – score 2–4; severe – score ≥5.

- As the disease worsens the stridor becomes both inspiratory and expiratory and present at rest. Signs of respiratory distress become more marked and hypoxaemia can occur.
- A chest X-ray may show sub-glottic narrowing, distention of hypopharynx and tapering of trachea (Steeple sign).
- The differential diagnosis is with epiglottitis, which usually has a more rapid onset, the child is more toxic, usually sitting and older.
- The severity of croup can be assessed using a croup score but this should not replace clinical judgement. The trend is more important than the actual score (Table 11.6).

Treatment
- Initially supportive in a calm atmosphere with gentle handling.
- Humidified O_2 with saturation monitoring should be provided – keep SaO_2 >90%.

RESPIRATORY DISEASE

11

- Adrenaline can be given via a nebuliser (0.5 ml/kg of 1:1000 adrenaline to a maximum of 5 ml). Can be repeated 3 hourly. This will give temporary relief for up to 2 h. Indications include deterioration, pre-intubation (facilitates inhalational anaesthesia), and prior to transport.

- Steroids – reduce the need for intubation in viral croup and reduce the duration of ventilation. A loading dose of 0.6 mg/kg of dexamethasone (max 10 mg) then 0.15 mg/kg 6 hourly. The steroids can be given orally, IM, IV or nebulised depending on the severity of the croup.

- Antibiotics – only for bacterial croup.

- Helium – Helium is a low density inert gas. When substituted for nitrogen in the inspired gas flow, the force required to move gas through the airways in decreased. Helium-oxygen mixtures have been shown to improve symptoms refractory to nebulised adrenaline temporarily.

Epiglottitis

- Epiglottitis is a severe life threatening infection of the epiglottis and surrounding tissues.

- While epiglottitis occurs most commonly between 2 and 7 years of age it can occur in adults and infants. The causative organism is most commonly *Haemophilus influenzae* type B. This causes a supraglottic obstruction with a rapid (3–6 h) onset with a toxic looking child. Usually the child will be sitting up, drooling with a muffled or gutteral respiratory noise. The child may be reluctant to speak or swallow and be pyrexial (>39°C).

- The diagnosis is made from the history and clinical signs. It is important to keep the child as calm as possible as airway obstruction can be precipitated by distress, e.g. IV insertion.

Management

- As the airway is in immediate danger, senior help should be sought rapidly. Consultants in anaesthesia/ICU and ENT surgeon will be needed as intubation can be very difficult.

- The child should be nursed where they are most comfortable and transferred to the operating theatre for intubation. Following a gaseous induction, intubation should be attempted, if unsuccessful a needle cricothyroidotomy followed by a tracheostomy should be performed to secure the airway. Often the most difficult time of induction of anaesthesia is during moving the child from the upright position on his or her mother's knee to the lying down position for intubation, as the epiglottis can fall back and obstruct the laryngeal inlet. Maintaining continuous positive airway pressure (CPAP) may help. Induction of anaesthesia takes longer than expected due to the narrow airway. Laryngoscopy should demonstrate a cherry red oedematous epiglottis which may prevent visualisation of the vocal cords and trachea.

- After securing the airway IV access should be obtained and blood cultures, U + E and FBC and glucose samples sent for analysis. Throat swabs should also be sent.
- Cefotaxime (150 mg/kg/day) or chloramphenicol (50 mg/kg/day) should be started intra-venously.
- Usually the child can be extubated after 24–36 h and will have fully recovered within 5 days.
- An algorithm for the management of acute epiglottitis is shown in Figure 11.1.

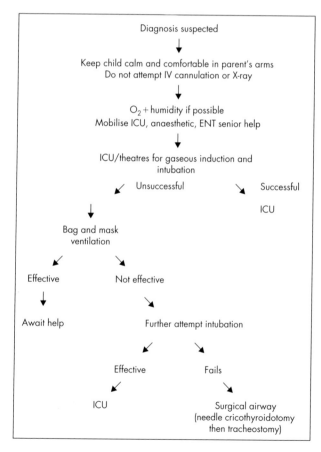

Figure 11.1 Algorithm for the management of acute epiglottitis

RESPIRATORY DISEASE

11

Lower airway illnesses
Asthma
Asthma still kills in the UK.

Incidence
The incidence of asthma is increasing, and hence the admissions to intensive care with life threatening asthma is also likely to increase. Boys have a higher incidence of asthma than girls.

Pathophysiology
Asthma is a disease in which air becomes trapped due to inflammation of the lower airways. It follows that expiration cannot occur fully and respiratory distress can ensue. In the toddler the process can be rapid despite optimal treatment.

Asthma in children is usually associated with a specific allergy (e.g. house dust mite or pets) and is a disease of exacerbations with variable symptoms between exacerbations. Many exacerbations have no identifiable precipitating factor but some may be associated with allergen exposure, infections, exercise, emotional state, environmental pollution and weather systems.

The pathological process consists of thickening of the basement membrane, eosinophilic infiltration, hypertrophy of the mucous glands and submucosal smooth muscle but with normal alveoli and remains despite the child being asymptomatic.

Differential diagnosis
- Acute infections: croup, epiglottitis, bronchiolitis and bronchopneumonia
- Aspiration of foreign body
- Congenital malformations: laryngotracheomalacia, anomalous subclavian artery syndrome (vascular ring), vocal cord paralysis and tracheal or bronchial stenosis

Assessment of severity
In assessing the severity of an acute exacerbation of asthma it is important to note the acute history including duration of symptoms, what treatment has already been given and to what effect. The course of previous exacerbations including any admissions to hospital, HDU or ICU should also be ascertained.

On examination respiratory rate and wheeze can be poor indicators of severity. The ability to speak, the use of accessory muscles and the presence of pulsus paradoxus (difference between systolic pressures in inspiration and expiration) greater than 20 mmHg are better indicators.

Table 11.7 Features of severe asthma

- Unable to feed or talk
- Use of accessory respiratory muscles and obvious recession
- High respiratory rate (typically >50 breaths per minute)
- High pulse rate (typically >140 bpm)
- Peak expired flow rate (PEFR) <50% of expected

Table 11.8 Features of life threatening asthma

- Reduced conscious level/agitation
- Features of exhaustion
- Silent chest/poor respiratory effort
- Reduced SaO_2 in air

The accurate use of peak expiratory flow meters will depend upon the age of the patient and the severity of the disease.

Arterial hypoxaemia and reduced SaO_2 on air are indicators of severe or life threatening asthma (Table 11.7 and 11.8).

Initial management
- Provide high concentration oxygen via a mask with a reservoir bag
- Commence nebulised β_2 agonists such as salbutamol (hourly or continuously if needed) and corticosteroids orally unless vomiting
- If the asthma does not respond to these measures then add in nebulised ipratropium 6 hourly
- Intra-venous aminophylline or salbutamol may need to be used in severe cases. An IV bolus of 15 µg/kg of salbutamol may aid the nebulised salbutamol to reach underventilated areas of the lung.
- Intra-venous aminophylline bolus, followed by infusion may be useful if the nebulisers are not fully effective
- Steroids act by increasing the number of β receptors and by reversing the down-regulation of the existing receptors
- This process takes a minimum of 4–6 h to occur
- Volatile anaesthetic agents halothane and isoflurane are potent bronchodilators
- Use of magnesium sulphate by loading dose 60–70 µg/kg followed by an infusion 20–40 µg/kg/h has been shown to be useful. Care with hypotension. Magnesium levels need monitoring.

If the child still has signs of life threatening asthma (see table above) then intubation and ventilation may be considered.

Criteria for intubation
The aim of treatment is to try and avoid ventilation because of the difficulty of ventilating these patients and the risks of air leaks.

RESPIRATORY DISEASE

11

The criteria for intubation and ventilation are mainly clinical:

- Respiratory arrest
- Signs of respiratory exhaustion
- Reduced breath sounds or a 'quiet' chest
- Reduced mental status – lethargy, agitation, coma, convulsions

Arterial blood gases can be helpful in assessing response to treatment and the onset of exhaustion. Usually the $PaCO_2$ will be below normal but a rising $PaCO_2$ may indicate deterioration. Persistent hypoxaemia and cyanosis refractory to oxygen therapy are poor prognostic indicators.

- Intubation should be by a rapid sequence induction following pre-oxygenation.
- Ketamine has been used as it is a bronchodilator and may help reduce the fall in blood pressure that is often seen during induction.
- The hypotension is due to a combination of high intra-thoracic pressures reducing venous return and a relative hypovolaemia. Treatment is with a rapid fluid bolus.
- Continued neuro-muscular relaxation may be necessary to reduce airway pressures during ventilation and to avoid ineffective effort by the patient.

Ventilation

Aims are:

- Lowest peak airway pressure possible, low tidal volumes, long expiratory time, low respiratory rate
- Acceptable gas exchange – PaO_2 >9 kPa, permissive hypercapnia
- Minimal intrinsic positive end expiratory pressure (PEEP) (the positive airway pressure due to air trapping in distal airways)

Although no one mode of ventilation has been shown to be better, pressure control ventilation provides some protection against barotrauma. It should be noted that as compliance will change tidal volumes will not be constant.

Complications of ventilation

- Pneumothoraces and other air leaks
- Hypoxia

Bronchiolitis

Bronchiolitis is an acute infectious, inflammatory disease of both upper and lower airways. It is the commonest, serious respiratory infection in childhood. 2–3% of all infants are admitted to hospital each year. About 80% of admissions for bronchiolitis are in the first year of life, and 50% are in the second, third and fourth months of life. Admissions prior to this are rare, presumably due to trans-placental transfer of maternal IgA giving protection.

Serious infections may be mediated by IgE antibodies which cause a Type 1 allergic reaction as part of a complex immune mechanism.

Aetiology

Respiratory syncytial virus (RSV) is isolated in approximately 75% of children, from naso-pharyngeal aspirate. Other pathogens implicated include the parainfluenzae virus types 1, 2 and 3, influenza virus, adenovirus 1, 2 and 5 and mycoplasma. Boys are more commonly affected and more often hospitalised. Prematurity, low birth weight, lower socio-economic status, parental smoking, absence of breast feeding increase the incidence of bronchiolitis while pre-existing chronic lung disease and congenital heart disease increase the risk of respiratory failure. Bronchiolitis is very contagious with viral shedding occurring up to 21 days following the onset of symptoms.

Symptoms and signs
- Fever and a clear nasal discharge precede a dry cough and breathlessness. Wheezing is common and feeding difficulties usually cause hospitalisation. The patient is usually tachypnoeic with respiratory recession.
- On auscultation wheeze and inspiratory crackles may be heard.
- The respiratory pattern may be irregular and there may be recurrent apnoeas. Apnoeas occur in about 20% of hospitalised patients and are more common in premature infants born at less than 32 weeks gestation.
- The apnoeas require intubation and ventilation in about 10% of these patients.
- A tachycardia of 140–200 beats/min occurs and the infant may appear pale or cyanosed.
- The degree of hypoxia is the best indicator of severe illness and often corresponds to the tachypnoea.
- The chest X-ray shows a hyperinflated chest with flattened diaphragms and air trapping.
- There may be lobar infiltrates and/or atelectasis in up to 20% of patients, particularly in the upper lobes.

Respiratory syncytial virus can be identified by direct immunofluorescent antibody staining or an enzyme linked immunosorbent assay (ELISA) from a naso-pharyngeal aspirate (NPA).

Clinical course

The majority of children will recover from the acute illness within 2 weeks, but coughing may persist for several weeks. 1–2% of patients will require intubation and ventilation, usually because of recurrent apnoeas, exhaustion and/or respiratory failure.

RESPIRATORY DISEASE

Between 20 and 50% of children develop a recurrent wheeze and cough over the next 3–5 years. Rarely there is severe permanent damage to the airways, bronchiolitis obliterans.

Management
- The main treatment for bronchiolitis is oxygen therapy and fluid replacement.
- Monitoring should include pulse oximetry, fluid intake and output, apnoea alarm and temperature especially in the small infant.
- Oxygen should be humidified and can be delivered into a headbox, via nasal CPAP or by mechanical ventilation.
- The inspired oxygen concentration should be sufficient to ensure a saturation of >93%.
- There is no convincing evidence to recommend the use of bronchodilators, corticosteroids or antibiotics. The wheeze is due to secretions not smooth muscle constriction.
- Nebulised and subcutaneous adrenaline have been shown to improve oxygenation and clinical signs compared with placebo.
- Ribavirin is an anti-viral agent which, when given by nebulisation, may help prevent ventilation in this group of patients. However, it is difficult to administer and has no evidence of effectiveness. It is used in high risk patients such as those with chronic lung or congenital cardiac disease in which mechanical ventilation is preferably avoided – it is not useful once ventilated.
- Mechanical ventilation should be at a rate slow enough to allow adequate emptying of the airways. The ventilator inspiratory time needs to be long enough to overcome the resistance to airway opening. High inspiratory pressures may be needed to help oxygenation. In infants with progressive hypoxaemia refractory to conventional treatments, high frequency oscillation or extracorporal membrane oxygenation should be considered.
- Those patients who are admitted to ICU often have different clinical courses:
  - infants who have apnoeas as their main presenting feature who require nasal CPAP or intermittent positive pressure ventilation (IPPV) for a few days
  - those who have pneumonia often with an up and down course with collapsed lung lobes on chest X-ray often with different lobes affected during the illness
  - those with a more severe pneumonitis who may need ventilation for 10–14 days

Pneumonia
Pneumonia in childhood may be caused by many pathogens, both bacterial and viral. The precipitating cause varies with age group (see Table 11.9).

Table 11.9 Infectious causes of pneumonia

Age	Causative organisms
Perinatal (<4 weeks)	E. coli and other gram −ve organisms Group B haemolytic streptococci Chlamydia trachomatis
Infancy	RSV Pneumococcus Haemophilus influenzae

Diagnosis

In younger children and infants non-specific symptoms may predominate such as fever, vomiting and obtundation. Cough and breathlessness with or without purulent sputum often occur. Pleuritic inflammation may result in chest, abdominal and/or neck pain. The classical signs of consolidation may be absent and may only be identified on X-ray.

Pleural effusions are reasonably common especially with bacterial pneumonia.

Treatment

Supportive for most non-bacterial pneumonia

- Chlamydia and mycoplasma should be treated with erythromycin 40–50 mg/kg/day usually orally.
- If pneumocystis carinii pneumonia is suspected co-trimoxazole 18–27 mg/kg/day IV should be prescribed.

Bacterial

<1 month	Ampicillin 75–100 mg/kg/day and Gentamicin 5 mg/kg od
1–3 months	Cefuroxime (75–150 mg/kg/day) or co-amoxiclav (40 mg/kg/day)
>3 months	Benzylpenicillin or erythromycin (change to cefuroxime or amoxycillin if no response)

This should be amended depending on local patterns of infection.

The general principles of treatment are similar to other ill children, i.e. hydration, anti-pyretics and ventilatory support if necessary.

Whooping cough

- Caused by *Bordetella pertussis*
- Diagnosed by characteristic 'whooping' cough
- Commonly develop secondary bacterial pneumonia
- Routinely vaccinated but herd immunity reducing due to reduced level of vaccine uptake

RESPIRATORY DISEASE

11

- Diagnosed by per-nasal swab
- Often have very high white cell count >20 mainly lymphocytes
- Treatment is supportive
- Humidified oxygen
- Chlorpromazine may reduce cough
- Ventilation as required
- Erythromycin reduces the length of infectivity but not illness

CHAPTER 12

CARDIAC DISEASE ON THE PICU

Congenital heart disease (CHD) – general points
- Incidence is 6–8/1000 live births
- More common in premature infants
- Causes are multifactorial and include known teratogens (diabetes, rubella, maternal alcohol) and associations with chromosomal abnormality (e.g. trisomy 21) or other recognised patterns of malformation or syndrome
- May be associated with a significant musculoskeletal defect (e.g. diaphragmatic hernia, exomphalos, tracheo-oesophageal fistula, imperforate anus)

Simple pathophysiological classification of congenital heart disease
Lesions causing primary left-right shunts
- Patent ductus arteriosus (PDA)
- Atrial septal defect (ASD) (Figure 12.1)

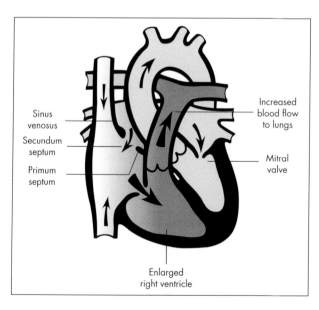

Figure 12.1 Atrial septal defect (secundum)

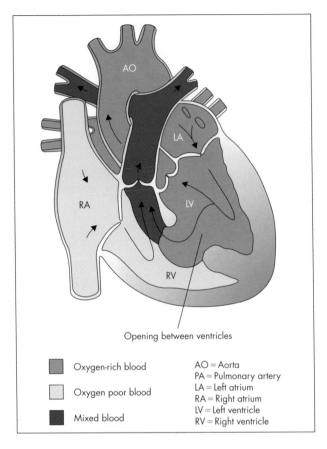

Figure 12.2 Ventricular septal defect (VSD)

- Ventricular septal defect (VSD) (Figure 12.2)
- Aorto pulmonary (AP) window
- Atrioventricular septal (AVSD) defect
- Systemic arterio–venous (AV) malformation

Lesions causing primary right–left shunts
The following lesions present with increased pulmonary vascular markings on chest X-ray

- Transposition of the great arteries (TGA), ± VSD
- Truncus arteriosus
- Total anomalous pulmonary venous drainage (TAPVD)

The following lesions present with reduced pulmonary vascular markings
- Tetralogy of Fallot (TOF)
- Pulmonary atresia ± VSD
- Tricuspid atresia ± VSD
- Critical pulmonary stenosis

Lesions obstructing ventricular function

These lesions may present with cardiac failure or cardiogenic shock.

Left heart
- Coarctation of the aorta
- Interruption of the aorta
- Critical aortic stenosis
- Mitral stenosis
- Hypoplastic left heart syndrome (HLHS)

Right heart
- Pulmonary stenosis

Shunts

- A shunt is a communication between systemic and pulmonary circulations and may occur:
  - outside the heart (e.g. collateral vessels, patent ductus arteriosus)
  - within the heart (at atrial, ventricular or great artery level)
- It may be a component of the congenital heart lesion or created to palliate it (e.g. a Blalock Taussig shunt).
- The magnitude and direction of blood flow across a shunt are determined by the size of the communication and by the relative resistances of the pulmonary and systemic vascular resistances.
- Shunting may be essential for survival (a patent ductus may supply the pulmonary blood in pulmonary atresia or the systemic flow in aortic atresia). Where there is complete or partial obstruction to a circulatory path, a communication at another level is essential.

Left to right shunts, general points
- Children are typically pink with increased pulmonary vascular markings on chest X-ray.
- Physical signs reflect the shunt volume (tachypnoea, reduced pulmonary compliance).
- Heart chambers enlarge and hypertrophy to cope with increased volume.
- Increased flow across a valve causes a murmur.
- Volume overload can ultimately cause ventricular failure.
- Sustained high pulmonary blood flow damages small peripheral pulmonary arteries.

- This can cause pulmonary hypertension, which may become irreversible (Eisenmenger's syndrome, in which flow through the shunt becomes R-L and the patient cyanosed).
- Initial management includes oxygen administration and diuretics (furosemide, amiloride).
- Intermittent positive pressure ventilation (IPPV) may be necessary to reduce the work of breathing and oxygen consumption, reduce ventricular preload, and prevent fatigue. Inotropes may be required.

Right to left shunts and cyanosis
- Pulmonary blood flow is maintained through a patent ductus arteriosus in 'duct-dependent' lesions.
- Prostaglandin infusion (2–20 ng/kg/min via a peripheral vein) is required to maintain the patency of the ductus.
- Side effects of prostaglandin infusion include apnoea and oedema. Endotracheal intubation and ventilation may be required.
- Unnecessarily high FiO_2 may encourage constriction of the ductus.
- Chronic hypoxaemia is associated with high haematocrit and raised cardiac output in order to maintain oxygen delivery.
- Thrombo-embolism can occur with dehydration or excessive diuretic therapy.

Specific lesions in CHD
Patent ductus arteriosus (PDA) (Figure 12.3)
- Shunt is at arterial level (PA and aorta).
- Closure of the ductus is a normal physiological adaptation to extrauterine life, and its persistence in neonates is a feature of immaturity (prematurity) or necessity ('duct-dependent' CHD). Abnormalities of ductal tissue may result in failure of the ductus to constrict in older infants.
- Magnitude of shunt depends on size of duct and relative resistances of pulmonary and systemic vasculature.
- A large L-R shunt may result in failure of a premature infant to wean from ventilation.
- Medical management encourages ductal constriction with cyclooxygenase inhibitors (e.g. indomethacin). Side effects and contra-indications include gastrointestinal haemorrhage, renal failure, intra-ventricular haemorrhage.
- Surgical ligation is via a left thoracotomy (after echocardiographic confirmation of normal cardiac configuration).
- Transcatheter closure with an occlusive device (coil or 'umbrella') is reserved for PDA in older infants.
- Untreated, a large duct can lead to progressive pulmonary vascular disease. Smaller shunts are at risk for endocarditis, aneurysm, calcification, and paradoxical emboli.

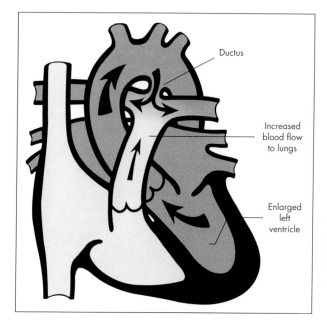

Figure 12.3 Patent ductus arteriosus

Transposition of the great arteries (TGA) (Figure 12.4)
- The aorta arises from the right ventricle and the pulmonary artery from the left (systemic) ventricle.
- Mixing must occur for survival, either through a septal defect or patent ductus. Percutaneous balloon septostomy may be necessary to encourage this.
- Approximately 50% of cases have an associated VSD.
- More complicated and rare forms of TGA are associated with pulmonary stenosis, or atrioventricular discordance ('congenitally corrected' TGA), or ventricular hypoplasia (tricuspid atresia). These require individualised surgical palliation.

Neonatal arterial 'switch'
- This is the preferred surgical option for uncomplicated TGA.
- It aims for anatomical correction and includes re-implanting the coronary arteries into the left ventricular outflow tract, and closing any ventricular septal defect.
- Difficulties arise when there are abnormalities of the coronary artery anatomy or compromised perfusion.

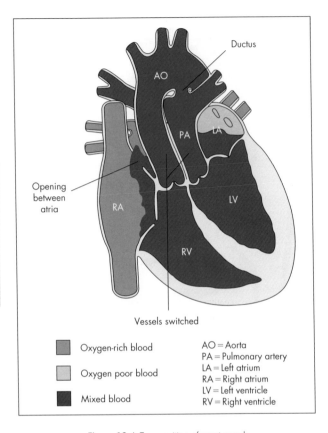

Figure 12.4 Transposition of great vessels

- There may be left ventricular dysfunction or ventricular dysrhythmia in the early post-operative phase.
- A 'late' switch is performed after a period of training of what will become the systemic ventricle, by placing a pulmonary artery band to obstruct the outflow from the left ventricle.

Atrial 'switch'
- This is a physiological correction, and less common nowadays.
- Surgery involves making baffles or channels in the atria such that venous blood returning from the body is diverted into the left ventricle, and then into the pulmonary artery (Mustard or Senning procedures).

- Post-operative atrial dysrhythmias are common.
- The disadvantage in the longer term is that the right ventricle eventually fails.

Coarctation of the aorta (CoA) (Figure 12.5)

Neonatal CoA

- In neonates, narrowing of the aorta occurs at or just proximal to the insertion of the ductus arteriosus.
- A more severe form is hypoplasia of the aorta itself (interrupted aortic arch).
- Systemic perfusion is dependent on a patent ductus arteriosus.
- Neonatal presentation is typically in cardiac failure, as the ductus starts to constrict. There can be rapid progression to cardiogenic shock with hypotension, acidosis and renal impairment.
- Resuscitation includes prostaglandin infusion, and IPPV and inotropic support in the sickest neonates.
- Surgical repair is by resection of the discrete coarctation and end-to-end anastomosis, or by using a flap of left subclavian artery to enlarge the aorta.

Late presentation

- The level of the coarctation is postductal.
- The clinical signs of murmur, differential hypertension, rib notching on chest X-ray, may be found on co-incidental medical examination.
- Collateral vessels develop which can cause troublesome bleeding at operation.
- Relief of the obstruction can result in rebound hypertension, requiring temporary vasodilator therapy or β-blockade.

Tetralogy of Fallot (TOF) (Figure 12.6)

- This is the combination of a ventricular septal defect and obstruction to pulmonary blood flow (usually at the outlet of the right ventricle, the infundibulum).
- There is secondary right ventricular hypertrophy and an abnormally positioned aortic outflow, which 'overrides' the ventricular septal defect.
- Blood flow to the lungs is reduced, but by variable amounts. Some children have few symptoms unless stressed, whereas others present early in infancy with cyanosis, particularly if the pulmonary arteries are also small.
- Hypercyanotic 'spells' are a result of spasm of the infundibular muscle and cause an increased shunt across the VSD to the systemic circulation (R–L).
- It is this *dynamic* aspect of the obstruction to pulmonary blood flow that accounts for both the intermittent nature of 'spells' and therapeutic interventions to curtail them.

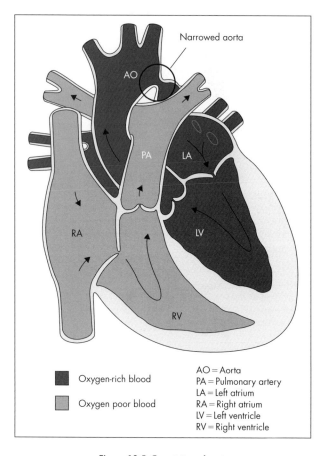

Figure 12.5 Coarctation of aorta

- Hypercyanotic 'spells' are detected by cyanosis, a reduction in end-tidal carbon dioxide concentration, and systemic hypotension (Table 12.1).

Surgically, a Blalock Taussig shunt may be fashioned if the pulmonary arteries are too small to accommodate primary repair.

- Definitive repair involves closing the VSD and enlarging the right ventricular outflow tract.

- Post-operatively, the hypertrophied right ventricle is relatively non-compliant and dysfunctional. This is more likely if a ventriculotomy has been performed.

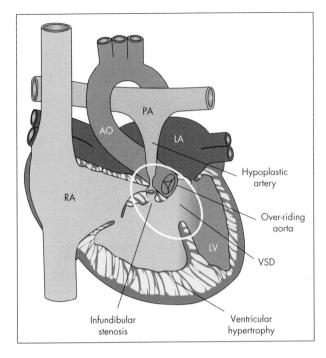

Figure 12.6 Tetralogy of Fallot (TOF)

Table 12.1 Management of hypercyanotic 'spells' in Tetralogy of Fallot

Hyperventilation with 100% oxygen to reduce pulmonary vascular resistance
Correction of hypovolaemia; colloid bolus
Elevation of the legs to increase systemic venous return
Administration of α-agonist to increase systemic vascular resistance, e.g. methoxamine, phenylephrine or norepinephrine by infusion
Analgesia and β-blockade (propranolol, esmolol)

- Double outlet right ventricle (DORV) is a variant of Tetralogy of Fallot in which there is greater than 5% aortic override.
- Pulmonary atresia is an extreme form of TOF, very variable in its severity.

Table 12.2 Features of the Fontan circulation

Blood flow from the systemic veins is directed to the pulmonary arteries

Cardiac output is dependent on adequate pulmonary blood flow

The pressure gradient across the lungs must be greater than PVR for forward flow

Factors promoting pulmonary blood flow are normovolaemia, avoidance of raised intra-thoracic pressure, spontaneous ventilation

Sinus rhythm maximises cardiac output

Anaemia should be corrected, to aid oxygen delivery

Anticoagulation is required

The Fontan circulation

Fontan – general points (Table 12.2)

- The classical indication is for tricuspid atresia with hypoplastic right ventricle.

- Univentricular heart lesions that are unsuitable for biventricular repair can also be palliated by a staged Fontan operation (Stage 1 SVC to RPA; Stage 2 IVC to MPA/LPA). An example is palliation of HLHS.

- An atrial communication (fenestration) is sometimes left, with variable potential for desaturation.

- High systemic venous pressures can lead to pleural and pericardial effusions, and ascites.

- Some patients develop pulmonary arterio-venous malformations, which cause cyanosis.

- Longer term, there is a risk of ventricular failure.

Post-operative cardiac management

- Paediatric cardio-pulmonary bypass (CPB) is similar to that in adult practice in that it involves full heparinisation, aortic and venous cannulation, non-pulsatile blood flow, membrane oxygenators, cross-clamping of the aorta, and myocardial preservation (usually cold crystalloid cardioplegia and topical ice).

- The systemic inflammatory response is also triggered.

- Paediatric CPB differs in that:
  - The prime volume of the CPB is large in relation to the child's circulating volume. Greater use is made of donated blood products, especially coagulation factors.
  - Greater use is made of profound hypothermia, including deep hypothermic circulatory arrest (DHCA). This facilitates surgical access to structures within the heart.
  - The magnitude of the systemic inflammatory response syndrome (SIRS) triggered by CPB is greater in neonates. Capillary leak is one of the manifestations of this.

Table 12.3 Common problems following CPB

Temperature instability	• Hypothermia if inadequately rewarmed • Hyperthermia with SIRS
Hypovolaemia	• Volume requirements increase with rewarming and vasodilatation
Hypertension	• Assess analgesia and sedation • Increased risk of breakdown of surgical suture lines and haemorrhage if untreated
Sinus tachycardia	• Assess cardiac output, volume status, analgesia/sedation, fever, seizures
Capillary leak	• Causes tissue and pulmonary oedema • Maintenance fluids are typically restricted to 50% of normal requirements in the early post-operative period

– Pericardial, pleural drains and temporary epicardial pacing wires are routinely placed. Left atrial and pulmonary artery monitoring lines are placed under direct vision through the surgical field.

Specific problems following CPB

Table 12.3 gives the common problems seen after CPB

Bleeding
- Heparin is reversed by protamine titration after cessation from CPB.
- The chest drains must be kept patent to allow blood to drain from pericardial and pleural spaces.
- Coagulation factors are diluted and inhibited by hypothermia, CPB, and transfusion of large volume. Platelet concentrate and fresh frozen plasma are often transfused particularly in neonatal surgery.
- Calcium should be administered with blood transfusion, and if ionised plasma concentration is low.
- An inhibitor of fibrinolysis such as aprotonin, initiated before CPB, can help reduce blood loss. It is reserved for patients at high risk of serious haemorrhage (e.g. repeat sternotomy, extensive suture lines, etc) because of the risks of anaphylaxis and concerns about venous thrombo-embolism.

Tamponade
- Is the external compression of the heart (usually by blood)
- Signs include elevated central venous pressure, low cardiac output, hypotension, tachycardia, dysrhythmia, desaturation
- Immediate resuscitation and treatment is required. The sternal wound is opened to relieve the compression. The cause is then identified.

Low cardiac output
- The causes of poor myocardial function post-operatively include:
  - The effect of SIRS

12

- Residual air in the coronary arteries after separation from CPB
- Inadequate myocardial preservation during CPB
- Dysrhythmia (may be exacerbated by electrolyte disturbance)
- Temporary pacing is required for symptomatic brady-dysrhythmia
- Lactate levels may be elevated

Pulmonary hypertensive crisis

- Defined as a sudden change in pulmonary vascular resistance, such that pulmonary blood flow is reduced and there is severe desaturation and hypotension.
- Susceptible patients are those undergoing repair of lesions with large L-R shunts, or obstructed pulmonary venous drainage.
- Initial management is hyperventilation with high FiO_2.
- Specific therapies aim to reduce PVR.
- Inhaled nitric oxide, a specific pulmonary vasodilator, is effective in some patients.
- Prostacyclin and sodium nitroprusside produce both pulmonary and systemic vasodilatation.

Renal dysfunction

- Diuresis is normal following CPB (hypokalaemia can result, particularly with concomitant diuretic therapy).
- Acute renal failure is more likely in lesions that have involved obstructed systemic blood flow, or prolonged surgery. Recovery is usually complete once the cause is reversed.
- Temporary peritoneal dialysis may be required.
- This causes less respiratory disturbance in neonates and small infants if a continuous cross-flow method is used, avoiding a dwell cycle and abdominal distension.

Neurological injury

- Damage to the recurrent laryngeal and phrenic nerves are recognised complications of surgery in the chest (producing vocal cord palsy and diaphragmatic paralysis, respectively). Recovery is usual, although occasionally diaphragmatic plication is required to assist weaning from IPPV.
- Focal neurological injury and seizures can occur as a result of embolism (air, thrombus), particularly if there is communication between the systemic and pulmonary circulations (paradoxical embolism).
- Global ischaemic damage is a complication of CPB with low perfusion pressure or inadequate temperature control. Periods of DHCA are usually limited to the minimum required to effect surgical repair whilst providing some degree of neuro-protection at low temperatures.
- Ischaemia of the spinal cord occurs with prolonged cross-clamping of the aorta. It is a recognised complication of late repair of coarctation of the aorta.

CHAPTER 13

DYSRHYTHMIAS AND MYOCARDIAL DISEASE

Dysrhythmias

- Commonly observed in critically ill children
- Dysrhythmias which may not be a problem in the healthy child may compromise the critically ill one (Table 13.1 and 13.2)
- With increasing age, the heart rate decreases with an increase in stroke volume

Bradycardias

Asystole and pulseless electrical activity are emergency situations and have been discussed in Chapter 6.

Sinus bradycardia
Causes of this include:

- Sinus dysrhythmia with respiration
- Sinus arrest or exit block can cause sick sinus syndrome

Table 13.1 Causes of cardiac dysrhythmias

Primary rhythm disturbances
- Paroxysmal supraventricular tachycardia
- Re-entry tachycardias
- Congenital AV block
- Congenital long QT syndrome

Secondary rhythm disturbances
- Post-operative dysrhythmias
  - Junctional ectopic tachycardia
  - AV block
  - Primary atrial tachycardia
  - Ventricular dysrhythmias
  - Sick sinus syndrome
- Metabolic derangements
  - Electrolyte disturbances
  - Endocrine causes
  - CNS injury
  - Hypothermia, hyperthermia
  - Hypoxia
  - Acute myocardial infarction
- Toxic
  - Tricyclic anti-depressants
  - Digoxin
  - Aminophylline
- Infections
  - Endocarditis, myocarditis
- Myocardial contusion from trauma

13

Table 13.2 Types of dysrhythmia

Bradycardia
- Sinus bradycardia
- Second degree AV block
- Third degree AV block
- Atrial, junctional or ventricular escape rhythms
- Asystole

Tachycardia
- Supraventricular tachycardias
- AV reciprocating tachycardias
- Re-entry tachycardias
- Atrial flutter or fibrillation
- Junctional ectopic tachycardia

Ventricular tachycardias
- Premature ventricular complexes (ventricular ectopics)
- Ventricular tachycardia
- Ventricular fibrillation

- Vagal episodes, e.g. with syncope
- Parasympathetic stimulation (vagus) may lead to bradycardia due to:
  - Hypoxia
  - Apnoea
  - Nasopharyngeal suctioning
  - Endotracheal suctioning
  - Intubation
- Raised intra-cranial pressure
- Sick sinus syndrome following cardiac surgery, myocarditis, cardiomyopathy or ischaemia
- Oversedation

Conduction abnormalities

First degree heart block occurs when all atrial impulses are conducted to the ventricles but with a prolonged P-R interval. Rhythm is regular.

Second degree heart block occurs when not all impulses are transmitted to the ventricles. These are divided into:

- Mobitz Type I block (Wenckebach phenomenon). The P-R interval gradually increases until an impulse is not conducted and a ventricular complex does not occur. This is due to a conduction delay within the AV node.

- Mobitz Type II block. This is characterised by the sudden drop of an atrial impulse without the increasing length of the P-R interval. QRS morphology may vary. Usually due to a conduction defect in the His conduction system. May progress to complete heart block.

- Complete or third degree heart block means that there is no conduction between the atria and ventricles. It is the commonest form of brady-dysrhythmia in childhood.

Treatment
- Correct possible cause
- Treatment of raised intra-cranial pressure
- Correct hypotension and hypoperfusion
- Use of atropine or isoproterenol (isoprenaline)
- Cardiac pacing may be required

Tachydysrhythmias
Sinus tachycardia
This may be due to many causes:
- illness
- fever
- hypovolaemia
- pain
- distress and anxiety
- certain drugs, e.g. inotropes, aminophylline

Supraventricular tachycardia
- Tachycardias with rate greater than 200 bpm
- Usually due to re-entry phenomenon via an accessory pathway
- Often present with congestive cardiac failure, can have chest pain or irritability
- May present with normal blood pressure
- Can be confused with other causes of tachycardia with low cardiac output, e.g. fever, septic shock
- ECG shows regular rates in excess of 150 bpm and can reach 300 bpm (commonly 200–250 bpm)
- ECG complex demonstrates normal QRS morphology, but P wave morphology may be abnormal
- Table 13.3 details treatment options

Atrial fibrillation
- Rapid chaotic depolarisation of multiple atrial foci leading to ineffective atrial contraction with a variable ventricular rate which is irregularly irregular
- Causes include:
  - Rheumatic heart disease
  - Mitral valve disease
  - Atrial septal defects
  - Ebstein's anomaly

DYSRHYTHMIAS AND
MYOCARDIAL DISEASE

13

Table 13.3 Treatment of SVT

- ABC with oxygenation
- Vagal manoeuvres:
  - Carotid sinus massage and the valsalva manoeuvre can be attempted
  - Diving reflex through iced water to head or face. Care as bradycardia or asystole can occur
  - Edrophonium 0.1–0.2 mg/kg acetylcholinesterase inhibitor
- Adenosine
  - Affects SA node and AV conduction
  - Also can be used for diagnosis of wide complex QRS tachycardia
  - Has to be administered rapidly as it is metabolised by erythrocytes (half life 8–10 s)
  - Dose 50–250 μg/kg increased in 50 μg/kg increments
  - If the tachycardia responds and then recurs use the same dose
  - Action may be prolonged in patients with drugs that interfere with its metabolism or exaggerate its effects
  - Can cause chest pain, bronchospasm, can accelerate tachycardias via sympathetic stimulation
- DC cardioversion (0.5–2 J/kg) but anaesthesia may be required
- Pacing may be necessary
- Maintenance therapy with amiodarone or digoxin. Propranolol in Wolff-Parkinson-White syndrome (WPW)

- Cardiomyopathy
- Hyperthyroidism
- Pulmonary embolus
- ECG demonstrates absent P waves and irregular and rapid ventricular rate with normal QRS morphology

Atrial flutter
- Very similar to atrial fibrillation but the ECG demonstrates a saw tooth pattern at 250–500 bpm
- Causes include:
  - Congenital heart disease
  - Cardiomyopathy
  - Rheumatic heart disease
  - Mitral valve prolapse
  - Pericarditis
  - Wolff-Parkinson-White (commonest cause under 1 year of age)

Treatment
- Propranolol if WPW
- DC cardioversion or overdrive pacing
- Digoxin will slow ventricular rate
- Amiodarone for prevention once returned to sinus rhythm

Junctional ectopic tachycardia
- AV dissociation with ventricular rate (170–200 bpm) exceeding the atrial rate
- Post-op VSD, Mustard operation or Tetralogy of Fallot
- Myocarditis
- Regular rate with normal QRS morphology
- P waves can be seen after QRS due to retrograde conduction

Treatment
- Often difficult
- Correct metabolic and electrolyte disturbances
- Digoxin – may slow rate
- Paired ventricular pacing to rapid rate leading to effectively only output on every second beat
- Induced hypothermia (35–37°C)
- Amiodarone
- Propranolol
- Surgical ablation of ectopic focus

Ventricular dysrhythmias
Premature ventricular contraction
- Wide abnormal slurred QRS without P wave
- Can be uniform or multiform (multifocal)
- Possibly at risk of worse ventricular dysrhythmias

Ventricular tachycardia
- QRS prolonged
- Ventricular-atrial dissociation is often present
- Causes include:
  - Metabolic and electrolyte disturbance
  - Post-cardiac surgery
  - Myocarditis
  - Cardiomyopathy
  - Idiopathic
  - Prolonged Q-T syndromes
- Torsades de pointes is a variant of ventricular tachycardia in which the height of the complexes varies
- Occurs with anti-dysrhythmic drug toxicity, tricyclic overdose, hypovolaemia and prolonged Q-T syndromes

Treatment
- Depends on haemodynamic status
- If not shocked lidocaine (lignocaine) 2 mg/kg repeat if necessary

- Procainamide or phenytoin may be successful
- Magnesium sulphate may be successful in torsades de pointes
- Amiodarone may also work
- If compromised circulation or unsuccessful pharmacological response, use DC shock under anaesthesia if required

Cardioversion
Indications particularly in the patient with cardiovascular compromise include:

- Atrial flutter or fibrillation
- Supraventricular tachycardia
- Ventricular tachycardia
- Ventricular fibrillation

Adequate sedation or anaesthesia is required

Complications
- Superficial burns
- Bradycardias including sinus arrest and exit block
- Injury to staff

Pacing (Table 13.4)
Methods
- Epicardial wires placed at surgery preferably atrial and ventricular
- Transvenous wire
- Oesophageal – due to close relationship to left atrium but only really useful for atrial problems, e.g. overpacing SVT
- Transthoracic by placement via a spinal needle either subxiphoid or left fifth intercostal space onto ventricle
- Transcutaneous – chest and back electrodes, higher current required

Table 13.4 Indications for temporary pacing

- Profound bradycardia
- Conduction blockade
- SVT
- VT
- Escape rhythms
- Drug toxicity, e.g. propranolol, digoxin, verapamil
- Electrolyte disturbance
- Diagnosis
- Post-cardiac surgery commonly:
  - Tetralogy of Fallot
  - Transposition of great arteries
  - AV canal
  - Tricuspid atresia
  - Complex congenital disease with WPW

Modes
- Depends on whether fixed rate, demand or sequential pacing is required
- Can involve atrial, ventricular or both being paced
- Which method used depends on time and requirements, e.g. fixed ventricular pacing for the cardiovascularly compromised child requiring rapid pacing
- With tachydysrhythmias either slow atrial pacing is used to under-drive the arrhythmia or overdrive the rhythm with faster rates and abruptly stop the pacing allowing the return to normal rhythm to occur

Practical points
- May need a skin reference electrode if there is only one ventricular wire
- Start at an appropriate rate for the patient
- Check stimulation threshold and increase the current to at least twice this level for constant capture
- Consider dual chamber pacing if possible
- Check function daily

Complications
- Usually rare
- Failure to capture due to incorrect placement, displacement or myocardial damage
- Pericardial bleeding and tamponade usually at time of removal of surgically placed wires
- Ventricular dysrhythmias

Myocardial disease
Ischaemia (Table 13.5)
Neonatal ischaemic disease
- presents with tachypnoea, hypoxia, heart failure, ECG changes
- differential diagnosis involves echocardiography to exclude con-genital heart disease such as TAPVD or transposition of the great arteries
- creatine phosphokinase or troponin may be elevated
- treatment is supportive with oxygen, ventilation if required and treatment for shock or heart failure

Kawasaki Disease
- acute, febrile, mucocutaneous lymph node syndrome
- mainly affect infants and small children under 4
- no cause found but can occur in clusters

Table 13.5 Causes of myocardial ischaemia

Neonatal ischaemic heart disease
- Hypoxia
- Increased demand
  - Persistent transitional circulation
  - Pulmonary hypertension

Congenital heart disease
- Cyanotic heart disease (e.g. total anomalous pulmonary venous drainage, transposition of great arteries)
- Obstructive disease (e.g. aortic or pulmonary stenosis)
- Anomalous coronary arteries

Increased demand
- Catecholamine administration
- Head injury

Vascular disease
- Kawasaki disease
- Embolism
- Trauma

Thoracic trauma

Hypoxic due to cardiac arrest

- non-specific panvasculitis occurs
- endarteritis of major arteries can occur especially in the coronary arteries
- this leads to potential arrhythmias, myocarditis, myocardial ischaemia, aneurysm formation and coronary artery stenosis
- aneurysms resolve but can rupture and cause sudden death years later
- other findings include diarrhoea, aseptic meningitis, meatal ulceration, urethritis, jaundice, hepatitis
- diagnosis requires remittent fever, cervical lymphadenopathy, mucosal changes, erythema of palms and soles, conjunctional involvement, erythematous rash
- treatment includes supportive therapy and aspirin 100 mg/kg/day and then 30 mg/kg/day maintenance

Infections
Endocarditis
- difficult to diagnose especially as most intensive care patients have intra-vascular catheters which are prone to infection and positive blood cultures
- echocardiographic findings plus definite positive cultures needed to make diagnosis
- echocardiography of line tips is important
- blood cultures are important but may not be positive if the patient is already on antibiotics when a presumptive diagnosis may have to be made

- clots may need to be removed
- duration of therapy varies depending on organism
- prophylaxis for procedures which could cause bacteraemia is vital, e.g. for dental treatment

Post-operative
- about a third of all cases
- usually following valve replacement rather than other surgery
- early onset within 3 months has increased severity of clinical presentation
  - congestive cardiac failure and shock can occur
- may only present with a fever and positive blood cultures
- early onset usually coagulase – negative staphylococci, *Staphylococcus aureus* or less commonly gram-negative organisms
- late onset commonly streptococcal infection
- differential diagnosis includes pneumonia, urinary tract infection or meningitis, post-pericardiotomy syndrome, post-perfusion syndrome (CMV infection)

Catheter-associated infection
- diagnosis confirmed when infection is proven in blood culture and from the catheter tip
- catheter removal often necessary especially if candida is cultured
- antimicrobial therapy via catheter may be effective
- increased risk of endocarditis in patients with line infection and a catheter infection

Viral myocarditis
- enterovirus commonest cause, often Coxsackie B viruses
- spectrum from asymptomatic to severe disease with heart failure, dysrhythmia or sudden death
- late effects include dilated cardiomyopathy
- may be direct viral infection or antibody mediated damage
- fever, cyanosis, respiratory distress, tachycardia, congestive cardiac failure and ECG changes occur
- investigations include echocardiography
- treatment is supportive including bed rest, control of congestive cardiac failure, shock and dysrhythmias
- may need consideration for transplant

Cardiomyopathy
- hypertrophic cardiomyopathy is characterised by increase in ventricular wall thickness especially the septum

- can result in a gradient across the left ventricular outlet
- symptoms include dyspnoea, fatigue or exertion, chest pain, dizziness, syncope
- presentation with congestive cardiac failure, cardiomegaly or cyanosis is possible
- echocardiography demonstrates asymmetric septal hypertrophy and may show reduced ejection fraction and fractional shortening
- there is a risk of sudden death from ventricular dysrhythmias, especially if there is left ventricular outflow obstruction
- treatment is supportive and may include diuretics, inodilators and inotropes as appropriate
- treatment of the outflow obstruction may help
- consideration for cardiac transplantation may be necessary

Hypertension (Table 13.6)

Table 13.6 Causes of hypertension

Essential

Renal
  Acute renal failure
  Chronic glomerulonephritis
  Chronic pyelonephritis
  Hydronephrosis
  Polycystic disease
  Dysplastic kidney
  Renal tumours
  Collagen diseases

Vascular
  Coarctation of the aorta
  Renal artery abnormalities
  Renal vein thrombosis

Endocrine
  Phaeochromocytoma
  Neuroblastoma
  Cushings syndrome
  Primary aldosteronism
  Congenital adrenal hyperplasia

Miscellaneous
  Intra-cranial tumours
  Drugs, e.g. corticosteroids
  Guillain-Barre syndrome
  Porphyria

ICU related
  Inadequate sedation
  Recovery from critical illness especially treated with inotropes
  Withdrawal from sedation, e.g. withdrawal syndrome from
    opiate or benzodiazepine or rapid cessation of clonidine

Consider other possible causes:
- With tachycardia
  - Pain
  - Agitation
  - Seizures
  - Fluid overload
  - Drug effects
- With bradycardia
  - Raised ICP
  - Drug effects

Treatment
- treat the cause
- appropriate investigation
- use of anti-hypertensives depending on cause and situation, e.g. use glyceryl trinitrate (GTN) or labetalol infusion, nifedipine or atenolol by mouth

DYSRHYTHMIAS AND MYOCARDIAL DISEASE

13

CHAPTER 14

NEUROLOGICAL AND NEURO-MUSCULAR DISEASE

Pathophysiology

The brain is contained within a rigid box from about 3 months of age. An increase of one of the constituents within this cavity leads to a reduction of the others and then a rise in intra-cranial pressure. Insults to the brain can be considered as primary and secondary (Table 14.1).

Consequences of brain insult

- Trauma causes accelerating, decelerating and shear forces. This can lead to damage to blood vessels and intra-cranial bleeding. Sub-dural haematomas are most common. Surgical intervention may be required.

- Secondary injury is due to subsequent events commonly hypotension, hypoxaemia or both. This leads to reduced blood flow and reduced oxygen delivery. This can be worsened further by raised intra-cranial pressure. Further ischaemic damage can occur. Damage to the sodium-potassium pump leads to increased intra-cellular sodium and water and the development of cerebral oedema and potential cell death.

- Meningitis leads to inflammation occurring in the sub-arachnoid space. This can involve blood vessels leading to vasculitis. Infarction can result. Raised intra-cranial pressure and hypotension can also occur.

- The effects of status epilepticus are a combination of the effects of the cause, secondary insults occurring during the seizure such as hypoxia, hypoglycaemia and the effect of the seizure on the brain. Increased metabolic demands are usually met by increased blood flow. Seizures of more than 60 min may lead to permanent sequelae.

Examination of the nervous system

Initial examination of the neurological system is by using AVPU, posture and the response of the pupils to light. 'P' corresponds to a Glasgow Coma Scale of 8 (Table 14.2).

More detailed neurological examination uses the Glasgow Coma Scale (Table 14.3). This requires modification below the age of 5.

Examination of the pupils is important to assess the possibility of intra-cranial hypertension or a space occupying lesion. A unilateral dilated and unresponsive pupil is indicative of a possible intra-cranial haemorrhage.

Table 14.1 Causes of acute brain insult

• Traumatic	– blunt trauma	
	– penetrating trauma	
	– crush injury	
	– non-accidental injury	
• Cerebrovascular	– vascular malformations	
	– thromboembolic events	
• Metabolic	– hypoxia	– cardiac arrest
		– drowning
	– suffocation	– near miss sudden infant death syndrome (SIDS)
	– infection	– meningitis, encephalitis
		– septicaemia
	– metabolic	– hypoglycaemia
		– hypo or hypernatraemia
		– hyperosmolar states
		– hypothermia
		– hepatic encephalopathy
		– Reye's syndrome
		– haemolytic–uraemic syndrome
		– drug intoxication
		– poisoning
		– inborn error of metabolism
		– status epilepticus

Table 14.2 AVPU score

A – Alert
V – Responds to voice
P – Responds to pain
U – Unresponsive
Also examine pupils and posture

The unconscious child

Figure 14.1 gives an algorithm for the management of the unconscious child. Resuscitation is the initial requirement for early management. Subsequent management depends on history, examination and results of investigations (Table 14.4). Causes of coma are given in Table 14.5.

Status epilepticus
Status epilepticus is defined as a single or series of seizures lasting longer than 30 min without regaining consciousness between the seizures. Status epilepticus can be either generalised or focal.

Treatment needs to be instituted promptly as continued fitting may lead to neurological damage (approx 25%) or death (4–6%).

The cause and presenting features of status epilepticus in children vary considerably depending on age. In the newborn the features tend to

Table 14.3 Glasgow Coma Scale

	Over 5 years old		Infants under 5	
Eye opening	Spontaneous	4	Spontaneous	4
	To voice	3	To speech	3
	To pain	2	To pain	2
	None	1	None	1
Verbal	Orientated	5	Coos and babbles	5
	Confused speech	4	Irritable cries	4
	Inappropriate words	3	Cries to pain	3
	Incomprehensible sounds	2	Moans to pain	2
	None	1	None	1
Motor	Obeys commands	6	Normal spontaneous movements	6
	Localises pain	5	Withdraws to touch	5
	Withdraws	4	Withdraws to pain	4
	Abnormal flexion	3	Abnormal flexion	3
	Extension	2	Abnormal extension	2
	None	1	None	1

be more subtle, variable in presentation and to include apnoea. The types of epilepsy can be classified into generalised or partial seizures (Table 14.6). There are four main categories of presentation (Table 14.7). The major causes are given in Table 14.8.

Effects
Status epilepticus has an effect on most body systems particularly if not treated promptly. Table 14.9 details these.

Management goals
- Treat ABC
- Start treatment using status epilepticus protocol (Figure 14.2)
- Look for any metabolic or electrolyte disturbance and treat if found
- Look for other causes
- Prevention of seizure reoccurrence
- Treatment of complications

Investigations
- Blood glucose
- Electrolytes, renal and hepatic function including calcium and magnesium
- Blood gases including acid-base status
- Full blood count
- Other appropriate to illness

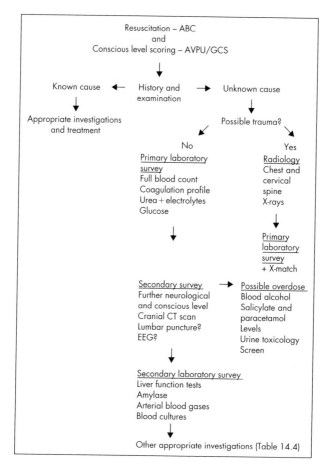

Figure 14.1 Algorithm for the management of the unconscious child

e.g. blood culture; anti-convulsant levels; metabolic, toxicology, viral titres
- CT scan may be appropriate when stabilised
- Lumbar puncture if raised ICP is ruled out

Supportive treatment
Intubation and ventilation may be necessary for:
- airway protection

NEUROLOGICAL AND NEURO-MUSCULAR DISEASE

Table 14.4 Possible investigations for unconscious child

Serum	Urine	CSF	Culture
Mycoplasma	Porphyrins	PCR for herpes simplex	Swabs
Viral antibodies	Organic acids	Viral antibodies	Viral culture
Ammonia	Amino acids	Culture and sensitivity	
Amino acids	Orotic acid		
Organic acids	Lactate		
Ketones	Ketones		
Fatty acids	Bile acids		
Triglycerides	Glycosaminoglycans		
Cholesterol			
Very long chain fatty acids			
Bile acids			
Immunoglobulins			
Lactate			
Pyruvate			
Acetoacetate			
Hydroxybutyrate			
Porphyrins			
Urate			
Minerals			
Vitamins			
Metals and metal binding proteins			

Table 14.5 Causes of coma

Cardio-respiratory arrest

Trauma
- Head injury
- Sub-dural, extra-dural haemorrhage

Infection
- Meningitis
- Encephalitis
- Overwhelming septicaemia
- Brain abscess

Intra-cerebral bleed
- Sub-arachnoid haemorrhage
- Cerebrovascular accident

Poisoning

Metabolic
- Hypoglycaemia
- Electrolyte disturbances
- Hepatic failure
- Renal failure

Status epilepticus

Cerebral tumour

NEURO-MUSCULAR DISEASE NEUROLOGICAL AND

Table 14.6 Types of status epilepticus

Centralised	Focal or partial
Tonic-clonic	Hemiconvulsion – hemiplegia – epilepsy
Tonic	
Clonic	Focal motor
Myoclonic	Epilepsia partialis continua
Absence	Complex partial

Table 14.7 Major causes of admission with status epilepticus (approximately 25% each)

Known epilepsy
Febrile convulsions
Acute insult
No known cause

Table 14.8 Main causes of acute insult causing status epilepticus

	Newborn	Infant	Child
Acute	Hypoxic ischaemia	Sub-dural haematoma	Trauma
	Intra-cranial haemorrhage	Trauma	Intra-cerebral haemorrhage
			Hypoxia
Infection	E.coli meningitis	Meningitis	Hypoglycaemia
	Encephalitis	Encephalitis	Encephalitis
			Brain abscess
Metabolic	Hypoglycaemia	Hypoglycaemia	Hypoglycaemia
	Hypocalcaemia	Hypocalcaemia	Hypocalcaemia
	Hypomagnesaemia	Hyper or hyponatraemia	Hyper or hyponatraemia
	Hyper or hyponatraemia		Liver disease
Genetic	Pyridoxine deficiency		
Malformation	Neuronal migration defect	Sturge-Weber	
	Chromosome abnormality	Neurofibromatosis	
Other	Toxins		Febrile convulsion
	Drug withdrawal		Idiopathic

NEURO-MUSCULAR DISEASE NEUROLOGICAL AND

- apnoea (may be treatment induced)
- hypoxia
- correction of acidosis
- coma and raised intra-cranial pressure
- to control seizures

It is important to remember that if muscle paralysis is used for intubation or maintenance of ventilation that this will mask the clinical

14

Table 14.9 Physiological changes during status epilepticus

Parameter	0–30 min	30–60 min	>60 min	Complication
Blood pressure	Increases	Increases	Decreases	Hypotension
Heart rate	Increases	Increases	Increase or decrease	–
Arterial oxygen	Decrease	Decrease	Decrease	Hypoxia
Arterial CO_2	Decrease	Variable	Increase	Raised ICP
pH	Decrease	Decrease	Decrease	Acidosis
Temperature	Increase	Increase	Increase markedly	Pyrexia
Pulmonary secretions	Increase	Increase	Increase	Atelectasis
Serum K^+	Increase	Increase	Increase	Dysrhythmias
Serum CPK	Normal	Increase	Increase	Renal failure
Autonomic activity	Increase	Increase	Increase	Dysrhythmias
Pupils	Dilated	Dilated	Dilated	–
Cerebral blood flow	Markedly increase	Increase	Increase	Cerebral bleed
Cerebral metabolic rate	Increase	Increase	Increase	Ischaemia
Blood glucose	Increase	Variable	Decrease	Hypoglycaemia

CO_2 – carbon dioxide; CPK – creatine phosphokinase; ICP – intra-cranial pressure; K^+ – potassium.

effects of seizures. The electrical effects will continue and thus EEG or cerebral function monitoring should be available.

Other problems
- Symptomatic use of fluids and inotropes as appropriate
- Maintenance of adequate urine flow to prevent the possibility of renal failure due to myoglobin excretion
- Hyperpyrexia can be reduced by using cooling methods and by stopping the energy production from fitting. If necessary use muscle relaxation following ventilation.
- Correction of metabolic and electrolyte abnormalities. In particular take care with hyperglycaemia in neonates.

CNS infections
Meningitis
This is a common disease in the paediatric population. There is an age related association with different causative organisms (see Table 14.10).

There is an increasing incidence of tuberculous meningitis. The incidence of meningitis increases following basal skull fracture, post neurosurgery, if there is a CSF shunt and in patients with immune deficiency from whatever cause.

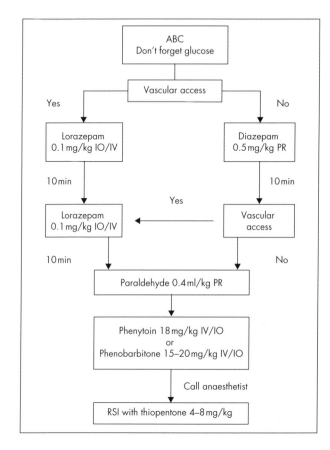

Figure 14.2 Treatment algorithm for status epilepticus

Table 14.10 Causes of bacterial meningitis with age

0–2 months	Group B streptococci
	Enteric (*E.coli*, Klebsiella, Proteus)
	Listeria
2–4 months	Group B streptococci
	Streptococci pneumonia
	Haemophilus influenzae type B
	Meningococcus
>4 months	*Streptococcus pneumoniae*
	Meningococcus
	Haemophilus influenzae type B (under 5)

NEUROLOGICAL AND NEURO-MUSCULAR DISEASE

14

There is evidence that intra-cranial pressure is increased and that there is a degree of hydrocephalus in most patients on CT scan.

Presentation
- Initial flu-like symptoms
- Fever, irritability
- Drowsiness progressing to coma
- Headache
- Photophobia
- Vomiting
- Loss of appetite
- Neck stiffness
- Seizures occur in 30%
- Remember to check for signs of septicaemia, e.g. purpuric spots in meningococcal disease

Focal neurological signs
- Sub-dural effusions
  - tend to occur at a week or later
  - commonest after *Haemophilus influenzae* type B meningitis
  - usually resolve spontaneously
  - indications for drainage include raised ICP, seizures, paresis, empyema
- Brain abscess
  - tends to present with worsening neurological signs and fever
- Hemiparesis or stroke

Assessment
- Neurological examination – may be difficult if ventilated and paralysed
- Ultrasound, CT scan or MRI of head for cause
- Doppler flow studies of major cerebral vessels
- Radionuclide scanning
- EEG

Prolonged or recurrent fever
- Fever persisting after 5 days or recurring
- Commonest cause is nosocomial infection but consider:
  - Ventriculitis
  - Sinusitis
  - Mastoiditis
  - Sub-dural effusions
  - Drug fevers

  - Sub-dural empyema
  - Disseminated infection, e.g. septic arthritis

Treatment
- Large dose of IV antibiotics:
  - Cefotaxime and ampicillin in neonates
  - Cefotaxime and vancomycin in older children
- Change antibiotics to appropriate when sensitivities from cultures are known
- Supportive treatment as required including management of raised intra-cranial pressure
- Steroids have been shown to reduce neurological sequelae of patients with *Haemophilus influenzae*
- Isolation of patient for 24 h
- Chemoprophylaxis for relatives or close contacts may be needed

Neonatal meningitis
- Most commonly acquired either at the time of delivery (strepto-coccal, *E. coli*, listeria) or hospital acquired
- Should be considered in the diagnosis of any unwell neonate and a lumbar puncture performed if appropriate

Viral encephalitis
- Infection of brain parenchyma following viraemia
- Prodromal viral illness including fever, lethargy
- Irritability and increasing coma
- Meningism, seizures, hemiparesis
- Poor feeding in infants
- Cerebral infarction
- May have spinal cord involvement
- Herpes simplex is commonest cause and only treatable virus (Table 14.11 and 14.12)

Investigations
- Routine septic screen

Table 14.11 Causes of viral encephalitis

Enterovirus	Adenovirus
Herpes simplex	Epstein-Barr virus
Varicella	Mumps
CMV	Measles
Rabies	HIV

NEUROLOGICAL AND NEURO-MUSCULAR DISEASE

14

Table 14.12 Differential diagnosis of encephalitis

Infection
- Meningitis
- Brain abscess
- Pertussis
- Lyme disease

Drug intoxication

Metabolic
- Reye's syndrome
- Hepatic encephalopathy
- Inborn errors of metabolism
- Uraemia

Presentation of cerebral cause
- Epilepsy
- Tumour
- Cerebrovascular accident (CVA)

Other
- Trauma
- Post-infectious encephalopathy

- Lumbar puncture
  - culture
  - pressure
  - PCR
- Metabolic studies
  - ammonia
  - organic acids
- Urine toxicology
- Imaging
  - ultrasound
  - CT scan
  - MRI – brain inflammation and oedema
- EEG
- Viral titres

Complications (see also Table 14.13)
- Cerebral oedema
- Raised ICP
- Seizures
- Neuronal destruction

Herpes simplex encephalitis
Neonates
- Diagnosis is often difficult. Approximately 50% have virus isolated from CSF in neonates, less than this in older children. PCR is often required.

Table 14.13 Complications of CNS infection

These depend on the age of child, organism involved, antibiotic therapy commencement and adequacy of treatment.

Acute
- Inappropriate ADH secretion
- DIC
- Septic shock
- Cerebral oedema
- Recurrent fever
- Seizures

Long-Term
- Mild to severe mental impairment
- Visual and auditory damage
- Epilepsy
- Hydrocephalus
- Behavioural abnormalities
- Hypothalamic disorders
- Hemi or quadriparesis

- Treatment with large dose acyclovir (4–5 mg/kg/day) for 2–3 weeks
- Can relapse if insufficiently treated

Infants and children
- Tends to be a similar illness as in adults
- Flu-like illness
- Fever, malaise
- Headache
- Vomiting
- Decreased consciousness level
- Seizures
- Neck stiffness
- Behavioural and speech changes
- Neonates may present non-specifically with sepsis and thus a lumbar puncture, if appropriate, should be a routine part of the investigation of sepsis in this age group
- Speed of onset depends on the organism

Lumbar puncture
- Lumbar puncture should only be performed if intra-cranial pressure is not raised and there is no coagulopathy. Complications include cerebral herniation or epidural or spinal haematoma respectively.
- Raised white cell count initially neutrophils then hyper-cytosis
- Xanthochromia and elevated numbers of red cells can occur
- Glucose level usually normal

- Repeat LP at 4 days may demonstrate a rise in viral antibody titre. A four fold rise is indicative of a likely organism.
- Convalescent CSF will often still give a diagnosis

Reye's syndrome
- Usually occurs shortly after an acute viral illness
- Most commonly in 6–12 year olds
- Associated with treatment with aspirin
- Much reduced incidence since its use has been limited

Presentation
- Nausea and vomiting occur usually 4–5 days after onset of the viral illness
- Altered behaviour, confusion leading to coma and death
- May develop decorticate then decerebrate posture with development of cerebral oedema
- Usually occurs within 2 days of presentation
- Elevation of transaminases to at least twice normal
- Liver histology consistent with syndrome aids diagnosis

Treatment
- Supportive control of especially cerebral oedema
- Early diagnosis and maintenance of blood glucose important
- No specific therapies
- High level of neurological sequelae in survivors

Pituitary disorders
- Inappropriate ADH (SIADH) secretion is defined as hyponatraemia and hypo-osmolality with normovolaemia. Also there is excessive urinary sodium loss and less than maximally dilute urine without renal disease.
- Treatment is fluid restriction with normal sodium intake
- Not all children with low sodium have SIADH

Diabetes insipidus
- opposite effect to SIADH leading to hypernatraemia and fluid depletion
- treatment fluid replacement
- DDAVP either by bolus or infusion to reduce urine output

Neuro-muscular disease causing respiratory failure
- Failure of the nervous system leading to reduced function of the muscles of respiration (Table 14.14)
- Treatment consists of treating the basic cause and supportive with oxygen, intubation and ventilation

14

Table 14.14 Neurological causes of respiratory failure

Cerebral	Central hypoventilation syndrome
	Drug intoxication
	Seizures
Spinal cord	Trauma
	Anterior Horn cell disease
	Poliomyelitis
	Spinal muscular atrophy
	Tetanus
Peripheral motor nerve	Phrenic nerve injury
	Guillain-Barre syndrome
	Intoxication, e.g. heavy metal, organophosphates
	Acute intermittent porphyria
Neuro-muscular junction	Myasthenia gravis
	Botulism
Skeletal muscle cell	Muscular dystrophy
	Congenital myopathies
	Myotonic dystrophy
	Inborn errors of metabolism
Electrolyte disorders	Hypo or hyperkalaemia
	Hypophosphataemia

- Comments on some conditions are given below:

Tetanus
- Severe painful muscle rigidity and spasms due to the neurotoxin, tetanospasmin from the organism *Clostridium tetani*
- This binds to presynaptic terminals of inhibitory neurones at the spinal cord level
- Allows uninhibited excitation leading to contraction of muscles leading to spasms
- The toxin binds irreversibly to the neuro-muscular junction leading to the need for new synapses to be formed for recovery
- Can affect laryngeal or respiratory muscles leading to airway obstruction or respiratory failure
- Incubation 3 days to 3 weeks
- Prevention by routine passive immunization
- Management is to prevent spasms by reducing stimulation and managing respiratory and cardiovascular complications
- Wound cleaning, antibiotics and supportive sedation, neuro–muscular relaxation and ventilation may be required
- Ventilation may be needed for 3–5 weeks

Poliomyelitis
- Severe form leads to widespread muscle paralysis and respiratory failure

14

- Respiratory failure depends on where the CNS is affected, e.g. central control of ventilation, phrenic nerve palsy, bulbar nerve palsy
- May lead to the need for chronic ventilation

Spinal muscular atrophy
- Autosomal recessive disorder
- Early presentation has a worse prognosis
- Progressive proximal weakness and hypotonia
- Paradoxical respiration occurs
- Present with failure to achieve motor milestones and recurrent pneumonia. Intelligence is usually normal.
- Diagnosis involves EMG and muscle biopsy
- Difficult to separate moderate and severe disease at presentation

Guillain-Barre syndrome
- Acute inflammatory peripheral neuropathy causing demyelination leading to weakness, paralysis and respiratory failure
- Associated autonomic nervous dysfunction including arrhythmias and blood pressure instability
- Often history of previous illness upper respiratory tract infection (URTI) or gastroenteritis or surgery 2–3 weeks previously
- Classically commences as symmetrical leg weakness which can progress proximally involving the diaphragm and pharynx
- Also have numbness and paraesthesiae
- May continue progressing for up to 2 weeks and followed by slow remission
- Areflexia is also present
- Treatment includes ventilatory support and plasmapheresis (daily for 5 days) or intra-venous γ globulin
- Most make a reasonable recovery of respiratory function

Phrenic nerve injury
- Most commonly due to trauma either during birth or cardiac surgery
- Presentation varies from mild to severe respiratory distress
- Post-cardiac surgery it may present as failure to wean from the ventilator with a raised hemi-diaphragm on chest X-ray
- Confirmation by fluoroscopy of the diaphragms
- Usually recovers post surgery 2–6 weeks
- Diaphragmatic plication may be necessary

Myasthenia gravis
- Chronic disorder with increasing tiredness of skeletal muscle during the course of the day

- Due to acetylcholine receptor antibodies
- ICU admission follows thymectomy or swallowing and respiratory fatigue
- Anti-cholinesterases will make diagnosis and help palliate disease
- Corticosteroids and plasmapheresis may be useful

Muscular dystrophy
- Congenital disorders leading to progressive respiratory failure
- Commonest is Duchenne's which is X-linked
- Gradual deterioration of skeletal and cardiac muscle with increasing age
- Present with pneumonia or post-operatively following scoliosis surgery
- Non-invasive ventilation increases length of survival

Critical illness neuropathy
- Critical illness neuropathy occurs in children particularly after severe sepsis and multi-organ failure
- Generalised weakness with respiratory muscle involvement occurs leading to slow weaning from the ventilator
- Can also occur in patients with status asthmaticus treated with high dose steroids
- Particularly associated with neuro-muscular blockade
- Hyporeflexia or areflexia occurs but usually spares facial and ocular muscles
- Diminished sensory function
- Prophylaxis should include the minimal use of neuro-muscular blocking agents, avoiding aminoglycosides at the same time as neuro-muscular blockage, correction of serum magnesium and phosphate and minimise steroid use
- Prolongation may also occur in liver and renal failure
- Recovery is usually complete but takes weeks

CHAPTER 15

GASTROINTESTINAL AND HEPATIC DISORDERS

Table 15.1 Main gastrointestinal problems on PICU

- Bleeding
- Illeus
- Diarrhoea
- Malnutrition

Bleeding
- diffuse, erosive, stress gastritis common
- presentation often as coffee ground or bright red blood in the naso-gastric aspirate or as haematemesis and malaena
- prevention important especially in conditions in which there is a high risk of erosions: burns, trauma, sepsis, acute respiratory failure, acute hepatic failure, steroid administration
- frequently contributes to death
- prevention includes early enteral feeding, sucralfate, H_2 receptor antagonists, antacids

Treatment
- intra-venous fluids including blood products
- surgical opinion may include endoscopy, ultrasound, arteriography, cautery to bleeding site may be necessary
- suppress further bleeding with enteral antacids, intra-venous H_2 antagonists
- if necessary embolisation by arteriography or operative intervention

Ileus
Causes include:
- post-operative due to surgery
- hypoxia due to shock
- effect of drugs (e.g. morphine)
- toxic megacolon
- intussusception

Diagnosis
- Abdominal distension
- Nausea and vomiting or increased nasogastric losses
- Decreased bowel sounds

- Dilatation of intestine
- Localised obstruction; may have abdominal pain

Treatment
Depends on cause but should include:
- Surgical opinion
- Nasogastric tube and decompression
- Avoidance of potential causes
- May require prokinetics, e.g. erythromycin for ileus

Diarrhoea
- Malabsorption
- Infection
  - e.g. colitis due to *Clostridium difficile*
  - bacterial infections, e.g. Salmonella, *E.coli*
  - viral infections, e.g. rotavirus
- Drugs:
  - Antibiotics
  - Chemotherapy
  - Feeds
  - Lactulose
- HIV

Treatment
- cause, check faecal culture
- treat symptoms, e.g. TPN
  - antidiarrhoeal agents
- avoid transmission to other patients

Malnutrition
Occurs frequently in long-term patients on the PICU causing a hypermetabolic state which is characterised by:
- Increased metabolic rate
- Increased sodium levels
- Water retention
- Breakdown of skeletal muscle

Treatment
Start feeding as soon as possible:
- Enteral feeding preferable
- Tube feeding by constant infusion associated with less reflux and diarrhoea
- Bolus feeding is however more physiological and possibly beneficial

GASTROINTESTINAL AND HEPATIC DISORDERS

15

- If enteral feeding fails start parental nutrition
  - needs central access
  - require appropriate mixture of amino acids, fatty acids and carbohydrates
  - should be commenced early if possible

Specific GI problems
Necrotising enterocolitis
- associated with prematurity, low birth weight infants
- no obvious cause known but probably involves hypoxic injury to the intestinal tract
- usually occurs within the first 3 weeks of life
- symptoms usually include abdominal distension, ileus, regurgitation and vomiting, malabsorption of carbohydrates, bloody stools
- abdominal X-ray shows fluid levels with intra-mural gas in the bowel wall

Treatment
- Antibiotics
- IV fluids
- Nasogastric tube and decompress for 7–14 days
- TPN
- Frequent X-rays
- Treatment of DIC using fresh frozen plasma (FFP)
- May need laparotomy and ileostomy
- Long-term may develop short gut syndrome which can lead to mal-absorption, need for long-term TPN, cholestasis and cirrhosis of the liver

Gastro-oesophageal reflux
- Common in neonates and infants and may not be symptomatic
- Causes apnoea, laryngospasm, bronchospasm, bradycardia, recurrent stridor, recurrent chest infections and possibly sudden infant death syndrome
- More common in patients with neurological impairment, e.g. cerebral palsy and after oesophageal surgery

Treatment
- thickened feeds
- increase gastric pH, e.g. omeprazole, ranitidine
- surgical – fundoplication with or without gastrostomy
- regurgitation and aspiration can occur during induction of anaesthesia and intubation especially with a potentially full stomach, e.g. after trauma

- cricoid pressure should help reduce regurgitation during intubation. However it should be removed if the patient is actively vomiting.
- treatment for pulmonary aspiration is antibiotics including traditionally metronidazole, physiotherapy and suction
- acid aspiration syndrome can lead to ARDS in the lung

Intussusception
- usually occurs in first year of life
- sudden onset on severe intermittent abdominal pain, with vomiting, and blood in diarrhoea
- dehydration and sepsis can occur later

Treatment
- Supportive, e.g. nasogastric drainage
- Reduction by barium enema or laparotomy
- May develop severe sepsis requiring antibiotics and intensive care

Hepatic failure
- Hepatitis C is more likely to cause liver failure than A or B (Table 15.2)
- Toxic causes include overdose of iron, paracetamol or hypersensitivity to NSAIDs, some antibiotics and anti-convulsants
- Raised liver function tests are common in intensive care probably due to multifactorial causes

Table 15.2 Causes of hepatic failure

Hepatocellular
Hepatitis A, B, C or D
Genetic and metabolic causes
e.g. α_1-antitrypsin deficiency
Wilson's disease
Neonatal diseases
e.g. rubella
herpes simplex
syphilis
Drugs and toxins
Obstructive
Intra-hepatic or extrahepatic atresias
Choledochal cyst
Cystic fibrosis
Cholangitis
TPN related cholestasis
Others
Hypoxia
Reye's syndrome

15

- Poor prognostic indicators and complications of hepatic failure are given in Tables 15.3 and 15.4.

Liver function tests
- The most sensitive test of liver function is the prothrombin time
- Bilirubin levels give an important indication of metabolism and are especially important in the neonate
- Albumin gives an indication of the synthetic properties of the liver but it is also dependent on other factors especially renal loss
- Most of the transaminase results have little correlation with the degree of hepatic failure particularly as falling levels may indicate loss of liver cells

Hepatic encephalopathy
- Worsens as the liver failure worsens
- Ammonia level increases with deepening encephalopathy but the actual level does not correlate
- Plasma levels of γ-aminobutyric acid (GABA) are raised in hepatic encephalopathy. This is an inhibitory neurotransmitter. See Table 15.5 for a clinical grading of hepatic encephalopathy.

Table 15.3 Poor prognostic indicators of hepatic failure

- Aetiology: non-A non-B viral hepatitis or paracetamol
- Age <10
- Severe encephalopathy
- Prolonged prothrombin time greater than 90 s
- Renal failure
- Rapid speed of onset

Table 15.4 Complications of hepatic failure

Encephalopathy
Cerebral oedema
Gastrointestinal bleeding
Ascites
Respiratory failure
Hepatorenal syndrome
Increased susceptibility to infections

Table 15.5 Grading of hepatic encephalopathy

Grade	Clinical features
I	Minor functional effects
II	Drowsy but rousable, confusion
III	Agitated to comatose with response to pain
IV	Unresponsive and unrousable

Treatment
- This is essentially prevention and supportive
- Avoid events which precipitate encephalopathy
- Reduce protein intake
  - Measures to prevent gastrointestinal bleeding
  - Avoidance of metabolic and electrolyte disturbance, e.g. hyponatraemia, hypokalaemia, hypoglycaemia
  - Prompt identification and treatment of infection
  - Avoid sedatives
- Supportive may include intubation and ventilation, oxygenation
- Treatment of cause
- Reduction of ammonia load by reducing protein intake
- Decreasing transit time with lactulose, use of neomycin to alter gut flora
- Flumazenil (GABA antagonist) may improve level of hepatic encephalopathy
- Charcoal haemoperfusion
- Liver transplantation

Cerebral oedema
- Main cause of death
- Develops as liver failure worsens in most patients
- Need to measure ICP as CT and MRI are not sensitive enough but care with abnormal clotting

Treatment includes:
- Maintenance of cerebral perfusion pressure with inotropes
- Avoid rises in ICP, e.g. coughing
- Reduce fluid intake
- Osmotic diuresis with mannitol and furosemide
- Reduce cerebral metabolic demand by control of seizures, hyperthermia and possibly the use of barbiturate coma

Gastrointestinal bleeding
- Many patients suffer this and 30% die from this
- Coagulopathy occurs due to a reduction in the synthesis of clotting factors V, VII and X
- DIC may also occur
- Stress gastritis is reduced by administration of H_2 receptor antagonists or antacids
- Portal hypertension leading to oesophageal varices can occur

Ascites
- Worsens respiratory failure
- Associated with portal hypertension

GASTROINTESTINAL AND HEPATIC DISORDERS

15

- Sodium retention and decreased oncotic pressure due to low serum albumin
- Treatment includes reducing sodium intake, slow diuresis using spironolactone

Hepatorenal syndrome
- Although frequently overloaded, often there is intra-vascular depletion
- This leads to a reduced renal output, an elevated urea and creatinine and a low urine sodium
- Treatment includes a fluid bolus, use of diuretics and measurement of CVP

Infections
- There is an increased susceptibility to infection due to bacteraemia from gut organisms, urinary tract infection, aspiration pneumonia, bacterial peritonitis

Pancreatitis
Causes
- Congenital anomalies
- Cystic fibrosis
- Amino acid dyscrasias
- Hyperlipoproteinaemias
- Association with hepatic failure

Clinical features
- Epigastric pain with radiation to the shoulder
- Tender abdomen
- Nausea and vomiting
- Decreased bowel sounds
- Tachycardia, tachypnoea

Investigations
- Raised serum amylase
- Hypocalcaemia
- Raised white cell count

Treatment
- Rest of pancreas by stopping enteral feeding, nasogastric decompression, using TPN
- Appropriate IV fluids and analgesia
- Complications may include abscess and pseudocyst formation

CHAPTER 16

RENAL DISEASE

Acute renal failure (Table 16.1)
- often part of multiple organ failure
- usually recovers without need for chronic treatment
- frequently multifactorial cause including sepsis
- defined as reduction in renal function with or without changes in urine volume
- anuria is an urine volume of less than 0.5 ml/kg/h

Physiology
- kidneys receive 20–30% of the cardiac output
- flow is autoregulated
- blood pressure is not a good indicator of renal blood flow because blood pressure tends to be maintained in hypovolaemic states while blood flow to the kidneys might be markedly reduced
- renal medulla is prone to hypoxaemia as oxygen consumption is high
- the blood flowing through the medulla has a low haematocrit
- the juxta-glomerular apparatus releases vasoactive substances to regulate blood flow to the glomeruli and hence alter the glomerular filtrate rate
- reduced blood flow leads to reduced oxygen delivery. In response to this, the juxta-glomerular apparatus reduces filtration. Fluid is retained and sodium reabsorption is reduced thus reducing oxygen consumption.

Table 16.1 Causes of renal failure

Prerenal/hypoperfusion	
Fluid loss	Haemorrhage, dehydration, septic shock, burns, surgery, diabetes mellitus
Decreased cardiac function	
Anatomical	Obstruction, e.g. urethral valves, tumour, blood clot, congenital renal disease, e.g. polycystic kidneys
Toxic	Myoglobin
	Haemoglobin (haemolysis)
	Contrast dyes
Immune	Haemolytic-uraemic syndrome
	Nephrotic syndrome
	Glomerulonephritis
Tumour lysis syndrome	
Infection	
Drugs	
Vascular	Renal artery or vein thrombosis

- medullary hypoxaemia is the main physiological effect causing acute renal failure

Prevention

Certain circumstances may be predictable:

- myoglobinuria/haemoglobinuria treat with aggressive hydration, increased urine flow by diuretics, alkalinisation
- tumour lysis/uric acid nephropathy
  - high fluid volumes to produce high urine flow
  - alkalinisation to prevent uric acid precipitating
  - xanthine oxidase inhibitors
- in general:
  - maintenance of adequate perfusion:
    fluid resuscitation
    inotropes
    blood
- treat the cause of sepsis

Management

- treatment of the patient for causative illness
- hypoperfusion needs appropriate treatment with fluids, blood and inotropes
- invasive cardiovascular monitoring
- appropriate cultures and antibiotics for sepsis
- appropriate operative drainage of septic foci

Fluids

- once acute renal failure has become established after resuscitation, fluid management involves replacing losses. These need to be measured.
- insensible losses are $300\,ml/m^2/day$
- temperature above 38°C leads to increased requirements about 12.5% per degree
- add measured losses, e.g. nasogastric aspirate, urine, beware diarrhoea

Electrolytes

- Hyponatraemia (see Chapter 8) (water overload)
- Hyperkalaemia (see Chapter 8)
- May have causes of increased potassium generation, e.g. haemolysis, tissue necrosis, acidosis

Renal replacement therapy (Table 16.2)

- method used depends on patient's size and condition and equipment and experience of staff (Table 16.3)

Table 16.2 Reasons for use of renal replacement therapy

Fluid overload, pulmonary oedema
Fluid removal to allow feed, transfusions, etc
Hyperkalaemia
Reduce acidosis
Endogenous toxins, e.g. urea, ammonia
Exogenous toxins, e.g. lithium, salicylate
Possibly removal of bacterial toxins, e.g. in meningococcal sepsis

Table 16.3 Methods available

Peritoneal dialysis
Haemodialysis
Slow continuous ultrafiltration (SCUF)
Plasmafiltration
Haemofiltration
   Continuous arterio-venous CAVH
   Continuous veno-veno CVVH
   Continuous arterio-venous with dialysis CAVHD
   Continuous veno-venous with dialysis CVVHD

Peritoneal dialysis
Advantages
- simple and easy to use especially in infants
- urea removal is gradual and steady

Complications
- may effect ventilation because of diaphragmatic splinting
- pleural effusions
- peritonitis
- catheter obstruction

Disadvantages
- respiratory effects
- less good than other techniques for fluid removal

Haemodialysis
- intermittent treatment
- removal of solute from patients' serum
- less useful because not continuous

Complications
- Hypotension
- Bleeding
- Embolism

RENAL DISEASE

16

- Catheter infection
- Disequilibrium syndrome due to osmotic shifts

Plasmafiltration
- the membrane contains larger pores than that for haemofiltration
- allows passage of molecules with molecular weight up to 3 000 000 Daltons
- thus endotoxins can be removed
- also lose albumin, immunoglobulins, protein-bound substances
- use in sepsis where large turnover of plasma can be achieved
- one plasma volume clearance clears about 50% of the plasma volume
- replacement fluid is FFP and albumin
- can be used intermittently in Guillain-Barre syndrome

Haemofiltration
CVVH
- primarily used for fluid removal
- allows removal of acid and potassium
- requires central venous access, blood pump, haemofilter, ultra-filtrate pump
- CVVH is pump driven and does not rely on patient's blood pressure
- anticoagulation required

Complications
- Bleeding
- Hypotension – decreased intra-vascular volume, increased inotropes
- Catheter infections
- Cooling can occur (an advantage in pyrexial patients but may mask continuing sepsis)

CAVH
- depends on patient's perfusion pressure
- needs arterial site for flow
- if hypotensive leads to low ultrafiltrate

CVVHD/CAVHD
- diasylate is pumped through filter to clear urea in addition to the ultrafiltration
- urea and creatinine clearance depends on diasylate flow

Haemolytic-uraemic syndrome
- multi-system disease of the microcirculation
- often accompanies *E. coli* enteric infection
- may lead to renal failure

- signs include:
  - – pallor, oliguria, tachycardia
  - – irritability, ataxia, tremor, behaviour changes
- investigations show anaemia, thrombocytopenia, uraemia, may have evidence of haemolysis

Complications
- Renal failure requiring dialysis
- Colitis
- Sepsis
- Myocarditis, pericarditis, pericardial effusion, ventricular dysfunction

Treatment
- plasmapheresis, dialysis
- supportive

Nephrotic syndrome
- protein loss in urine leads to hypoalbuminaemic oedema
- mostly caused by nephritis and treatment is by steroids
- oedema worsened by sodium retention
- prone to infections including peritonitis, pneumonia, urinary tract infection (UTI)
- raising the albumin level is probably only short-lived but with diuretics may establish a diuresis
- other treatment is supportive

Haemoglobinaemia
- caused by red blood cell lysis, e.g. post-transfusion reaction, extra-corporeal membrane oxygenation (ECMO), haemolytic–uraemic syndrome
- red blood cell stroma may cause mechanical obstruction in the renal capillaries
- treatment includes aggressive hydration and alkalinisation of urine flow with bicarbonate and carbonic anhydrase inhibitors
- mannitol and furosemide increase urine flow and may help the tubular obstruction
- exchange transfusion or plasmapheresis may lower levels

Myoglobinaemia
- following muscle injury and rhabdomyolysis including cardiac arrest
- diagnosis includes myoglobin in the urine and an elevated creatine phosphokinase (CPK)
- hyperkalaemia and renal failure may ensue
- treatment is alkalinised diuresis keeping the pH >7.0

RENAL DISEASE

16

CHAPTER 17

HAEMATOLOGY AND ONCOLOGY

Table 17.1 Haematological problems on PICU

Anaemia
Thrombocytopenia
Neutropenia
DIC
Sickle cell disease
Tumours including leukaemias
Bone marrow transplantation

Table 17.2 Causes of anaemia

- Abnormal red cell production
  Disorders of proliferation and differentiation
  Disorders of DNA synthesis
  Disorders of haemoglobin synthesis
- Increased RBC destruction
  Membrane defects
  Abnormal metabolism
  Mechanical destruction
  Infection
  Antibody mediated
  Hypersplenism
- Blood loss

Sickle cell disease

Causes of ICU admission include:

- susceptible to infection
- vasocculsive crises:
  - acute occlusion of vessels due to sickling
  - treatment includes oxygenation, hydration, analgesia and anti-biotics
  - acute chest syndrome. Symptoms include – cough, dyspnoea and chest pain. This can be caused by infection, pulmonary infarction or vasocclusive crisis. There is a variable course from mild pneumonia to fatal pulmonary disease.

Treatment includes:

  - antibiotics and analgesia
  - intra-venous fluids avoiding dehydration
  - exchange transfusion
  - heparinisation may be useful
- stroke – may need to control intra-cranial pressure

17

- may present with bony or abdominal crises
- acute splenic sequestration
  - presents with pallor, profound hypovolaemia and circulatory failure
  - treatment with fluids including blood

Leukaemias/tumours
- causes of ICU admission include:
  - septicaemia following chemotherapy with neutropenia
  - implanted line infections (including Candida)
- tumour lysis syndrome

Tumour lysis syndrome
- hyperuricaemia, hyperkalaemia, hyperphosphataemia
- may lead to hypercalcaemia and acute renal failure
- usually precipitated by cell lysis after commencing chemotherapy

Signs
Arrhythmias due to hyperkalaemia or hypercalcaemia.

Renal failure. This is in part due to urate and calcium phosphate deposition in the kidney. This leads to obstruction in the tubules.

Prevention of renal failure important:
  - generous hydration
  - prevention of formation of toxic metabolites – allopurinol
  - alkalinisation of urine
- haemodialysis may be required
- ECG monitoring

DIC
Many causes but gram-negative and meningococcal sepsis and major trauma the commonest causes. This leads to fibrogen consumption and microthrombi formation.

Signs and symptoms
- haemorrhage
- microthrombosis leading to organ ischaemia and failure including:
  - purpura fulminans
  - renal failure
  - confusion and coma
  - pulmonary and GI disturbance
- consumption of clotting factors and inhibitors of coagulation

Treatment
- underlying cause
- blood products, FFP, platelets, cryoprecipitate, Protein C
- the use of heparin has been advocated but shown to increase bleeding in adults

Bone marrow transplantation

The major complications after bone marrow transplant leading to PICU admission are detailed in Table 17.3.

Table 17.3 Complications following bone marrow transplantation

Pancytopenia
Infections
Mucositis
Chemotherapy induced drug toxicity
Graft versus host disease
Rejection
Veno-occlusive disease
Relapse

Pancytopenia
- for 2–4 weeks following chemotherapy
- possibility of opportunistic infection
- prolonged depressed T cell and B polymorph function
- G-CSF may reduce the time of this depressed cell function
- require irradiated blood products
- maintain platelets above $20\,000\,mm^{-3}$
- if bleeding maintain above $50–100\,000\,mm^{-3}$

Infection
- prevention better than cure including prophylactic antibiotics
- specific infections tend to vary with time post transplant
- fungi: candida, aspergillus
- viruses: HSV, EBV, CMV, RSV
- pneumocystis

Chemotherapy induced toxicity
- pulmonary toxicity important especially after bleomycin
- toxicity worsened by high FiO_2 and high airway pressures

Graft versus host disease (GVHD)
- due to T cells attacking the host
- affects skin, GI tract, liver and lungs
- acute insidious onset with fever, rash, diarrhoea, interstitial pneumonitis, nausea and vomiting

- chronic GVHD begins between day 100 and 2 years post transplant
- needs early recognition often by biopsy in sub-acute phase and aggressive immunosupression along with prophylaxis against fungal and pneumocystic infections

Veno-occlusive disease
- obliteration of small hepatic venules
- onset 1–3 weeks after bone marrow transplantation
- weight gain, hepatic enlargement, ascites, raised bilirubin may lead to encephalopathy
- treatment includes supportive treatment such as ventilation, fluid and electrolyte management
- repeat ultrasounds of flow in portal blood system helps with monitoring progress of disease

Solid tumours
Patients with various other tumours may well present to the PICU following major surgery requiring ventilation, management of major peri-operative blood loss or epidural analgesia. Some of the problems which may lead to admission for other reasons are given below.

Compromised airway:
- Cystic hygroma
- Laryngeal papillomata
- Intra-thoracic tumours

Compromised breathing:
- Intra-thoracic tumours
- Diaphragmatic splinting from intra-abdominal tumours

Hypertension
- Renal tumours
- Phaeochromocytoma

Cerebral tumours
- Raised ICP
- Reduced conscious level
- Loss of gag reflex, etc – posterior fossa tumour

Sepsis
- Following chemotherapy
- Line associated

Children with intra-thoracic tumours may present with stridor and a compromised airway. They are at grave risk of tracheal collapse on induction of anaesthesia and therefore senior anaesthetic help should be available if intubation and ventilation is required. It is preferable to attempt other methods to reduce the airway obstruction first, e.g. steroids, nebulised adrenaline, helium-oxygen inhalation.

17

CHAPTER 18

ENDOCRINE DISORDERS

Glucose metabolism

Table 18.1 Causes of hyperglycaemia

Stress response
Catecholamine response
Hypothermia
Dextrose administration
Diabetes mellitus

Table 18.2 Causes of hypoglycaemia

Deficient substrate
  Ketotic hypoglycaemia
  Inadequate infused glucose IV

Deranged endocrine balance
  Hyperinsulinism including infants of diabetic mothers
  Hypothyroidism
  Adrenal insufficiency
  Glucagon deficiency

Defective release from liver (inborn errors)
  Glycogen storage diseases I, III, IV
  Galactosaemia
  Fructose intolerance

Liver disease
  Hepatitis
  Cirrhosis
  Reye's syndrome
  Hepatic failure

Inborn errors of amino acid metabolism
  Maple syrup urine disease
  Proprionic acidaemia
  Isovaleric acidaemia
  Tyrosinosis
  Methylmalonic aciduria

Deficiency of fatty acid oxidation
  Medium and long chain acetyl CoA dehydrogenase deficiency

Drug-induced hypoglycaemia
  Insulin
  Salicylates
  Propranolol
  Alcohol
  Sulphonylureas
  Paracetamol

Diabetic ketoacidosis

Patient may present with:

- history (previously known diabetes)
- familiar history – polyuria, polydypsia, weight loss
- headache
- abdominal pain
- vomiting
- lethargy
- hyperpnoea

Can present with:

- profound shock
- coma
- respiratory failure
- dysrhythmias

Investigations:

- blood gases including pH
- electrolytes
- urea
- glucose
- osmolality
- ketones
- lactate
- calcium
- magnesium
- phosphate
- serum amylase (may be moderately raised – salivary isoenzyme)

It is important to monitor acid-base status, glucose and electrolytes frequently during the early stages.

Management

- ABC
- Fluid replacement is in three sections
- Volume replacement with 0.9% saline or colloid
- Maintenance fluid
- Fluid for dehydration
- Consider as if no more than 10% dehydrated
- Deficit should be given over 48 h
- Replacement fluid should initially be 0.9% saline until glucose has fallen to 12 mmol/l

18

Potassium
- Potassium needs to be given as there is large depletion of the intra-cellular ion
- Insulin will reduce plasma K^+
- Add 20 mmol KCl per 500 ml bag of fluid
- Frequent U & E estimation necessary
- Monitor ECG for hyper or hypokalaemia

Insulin
- Blood glucose will be falling because of the fluid replacement
- Use of continuous infusion is preferred
- Commence at 0.1 units/kg/h of actrapid
- If blood glucose falls too quickly ($>$5 mmol/l/h) then reduce infusion
- Switches off ketone production
- Reduce rate of infusion when glucose level falls below 12 mmol/l
- Preferable to increase % glucose delivered rather than stop the insulin infusion

General principles
- Keep close eye on fluid balance
- If concerned slow rehydration down and consider transfer to PICU

Complications (Table 18.3)

Shock – due to inadequate fluid replacement, need arterial, CVP and urinary catheter to adequately assess resuscitation

Cerebral oedema
- cause of mortality with poor outcome approximately 1% of admissions
- higher risk than in adults
- usually occurs in newly diagnosed diabetes often several hours after admission when all seems to be well
- symptoms include headache, reduced conscious level, bradycardia, papilloedema, fixed dilated pupils, occasionally polyuria due to diabetes insipidus
- theory is that rapid correction of fluid loss with reduction in high glucose levels leads to cerebral oedema due to the hyperosmolar state of brain cells
- may be direct effect of insulin on Na^+ and K^+ and water entering brain cells
- treatment involves the prediction that it may occur and therefore correct the fluid depletion slowly over 48 h
- if cerebral oedema occurs, intubation and ventilation is indicated

Table 18.3 Complications of diabetic ketoacidosis

Cerebral oedema
Pulmonary oedema
Dysrhythmias
Hypokalaemia
Hypoglycaemia (over correction)
Hypocalcaemia

- CT scanning and/or ICP monitoring should be considered
- mannitol may be useful
- outcome is poor therefore prevention is important

Hyperosmolar hyperglycaemic non-ketotic coma
- Rare in childhood
- Characterised by coma with hyperglycaemic dehydration without ketoacidosis
- Causes include lack of water, too much glucose or excess glucagon secretion
- Treatment fluid boluses for shock
- Care with insulin as blood glucose can drop very rapidly

Hypoglycaemia
- Consider as a cause of fitting, jitteriness and in all neonates
- Treatment is by giving 10% dextrose 5 ml/kg

Thyroid disease
- Thyrotoxicosis presents rarely to intensive care in children
- Symptoms are often insidious in onset
- Can be precipitated by infection, trauma, surgery, diabetic keto-acidosis
- Symptoms include hyperactivity of the sympathetic system nervousness, tachycardia, weakness
- Also auto antibody effects such as goitre and exophthalmos
- Thyroid crisis can lead to fever, tachycardia, dysrhythmias, abdominal pain, leading to hyperpyrexia, coma, cardiovascular collapse
- Associated with family history or other known associated conditions such as diabetes mellitus, Down's syndrome, Addison's disease and other autoimmune diseases

Treatment
- Supportive 'ABC'
- Fluids and electrolyte correction
- Treatment of pyrexia
- β–blockade (propranolol 0.01 mg/kg repeated until circulation controlled maximum 5 mg) and anti-thyroid drugs required

Hypothyroid

- Can be primary hypothyroid or sick euthyroid syndrome
- Commonest cause is non-thyroid illness causing depression of T3 and sometimes T4 without TSH elevation
- In adults it has been shown that correlation with severity of illness occurs but levels are difficult to raise with supplements
- Various drugs affect hormone levels

Adrenal disease

Phaeochromocytoma

- Catecholamine secreting tumour from adrenal medulla or sometimes within the sympathetic nervous chain
- Can be multiple or familial
- Effects are due to markedly raised levels of epinephrine and nor-epinephrine
- Sustained hypertension progressing to encephalopathy; cardiac failure can occur
- Can have paroxysmal episodes with palpitations, headache, flushing, feelings of impending doom
- Diagnosis is by urinary catecholamine metabolites

Treatment

- Surgical removal
- However, surgery may cause severe hypertensive episodes particularly during tumour manipulation
- α-receptor blockade needs to be instigated prior to β-blockade. Phentolamine and propranolol are used.
- Post-op the blood pressure may fluctuate. Hypotension can be treated with fluids and blood products.

Persistent hypertension may be due to further phaeochromocytoma tissue or another tumour.

CHAPTER 19

INBORN ERRORS OF METABOLISM

Can be admitted to PICU with:

Known diagnosis
- post-operative
- intercurrent illness
- metabolic imbalance

Unknown diagnosis
- neonatal
- change of diet or hypoglycaemia
- incidental finding

Children may have had perinatal diagnosis, e.g. phenylketonuria, galactosaemia.

Often presentation is non-specific (see Table 19.1). It may be confused with or present at the same time as sepsis. Family history is important.

Investigations
Initial

Blood sugar	FBC
Serum electrolytes	Clotting
Bicarbonate and acid-base	LFTs
Ammonia	Free fatty acids (FFA) and ketones

Urine for odour, acetest, organic and amino acids

Lactate

Other investigations
- Blood culture
- Amino acids, carnitine, creatinine kinase

Table 19.1 Signs and symptoms of inborn errors of metabolism

Vomiting	Acidosis
Dehydration	Hyperammonaemia
Hypoglycaemia	Jaundice
Lethargy	Hepatomegaly
Cerebral oedema	Cardiomyopathy
Seizures	
Ataxic movements	
Coma	
Respiratory distress	

19

- Urine culture
- CSF lactate and culture
- Keep sample of blood, urine and CSF for further analysis

If the patient has a metabolic acidosis:

- check if adequately resuscitated
- calculate anion gap. If >12 investigate cause of the acidosis as likely to be inborn error.
- ketosis and hypoglycaemia:
  - glycogen storage disease
  - gluconeogenesis defect
  - non-ketotic hypoglycaemia
  - fatty acid oxidation defect
- lactic acid and lactic:pyruvate ratios
- high lactate and high ratio is seen in:
  - anaerobic respiration
  - respiratory chain defect
  - mitochondrial myopathy
  - pyruvate carboxylase deficiency
- low ratio:
  - pyruvate dehydrogenase deficiency
- high levels with normal ratio:
  - pyruvate dehydrogenase deficiency
  - defect in gluconeogenesis

Specific groups of disorders

Urea cycle disorders
- hyperammonaemia
- no acidosis
- normal glucose
- specific disorders:
  - citrullinaemia, argininaemia, argininosuccinicacidaemia
- non-specific elevation of amino acids
  - ornithine transcarbamylase deficiency (OTC)
  - carbamylphosphate synthase deficiency (CPS)

Organic acidaemias
- hyperammonaemia (usually only around newborn period)
- relapsing course possible
- severe acidosis with vomiting and dehydration with ketosis
- may be difficult to distinguish from renal tubular acidosis

Lipid disorders
- usually present after a fast with vomiting and non-ketotic hypoglycaemia proceeding to coma
- may also have cardiomyopathy

Carbohydrate disorders
- galactosaemia may present with jaundice, acidosis, hypoglycaemia, gram-negative sepsis
- others may cause lactic acidosis

Treatment – general
- Supportive including antibiotics
- Dextrose for low BM
- Stop enteral feed. Give 10% Glucose IV.
- Preferable to add insulin if patient becomes hyperglycaemic rather than reducing dextrose concentration to stop protein breakdown and accumulation of toxic metabolites

Hyperammonaemia
If cause unknown give:
- arginine 300 mg/kg/day IV – reacts with ammonia to aid excretion
- sodium benzoate 500 mg/kg/day IV – conjugates with glycine
- sodium phenylbutyrate 600 mg/day IV – conjugates with glutamine
- carnitine 200 mg/kg/day IV in four doses per day – aids elimination of organic acids

Avoid alkalosis
- do not hyperventilate
- use bicarbonate if pH <7.2

If ammonia >500 μmol/l or >300 μmol/l with encephalopathy commence high turnover CVVH. Acute reduction of ammonia is important for outcome.

Other treatments
- CVVH may also be used for severe acidosis and in maple syrup urine disease
- Carnitine helps to excrete organic acids
- Specific treatments depending on diagnosis

CHAPTER 20

INFECTION AND RELATED ILLNESS

Meningococcal septicaemia

- May progress very rapidly with mortality of up to 50%.
- All patients with suspected meningococcaemia should be considered for admission to ICU and vigilantly observed for the first 24–48 h.

Clinical features

- Often preceded by a prodromal coryzal (flu-like) illness for a few days.
- Symptoms include: fever, rash, drowsiness, headache, irritability, convulsions, poor feeding, vomiting, and diarrhoea. Can present with or without meningitis.
- Rash may initially be absent or be preceded by less typical maculo-papular rash.
- Signs (neck stiffness, hypotension, coma) and the petechial non-blanching rash can develop rapidly.
- The course of the disease during the first 24–48 h can be extremely unpredictable.

Glasgow Meningococcal Septicaemia Prognostic Score (GMSPS)

- The GMSPS is a clinical scoring system that can be calculated rapidly and frequently and is used to predict severity. Score >8 indicates severe disease. Score >12 has a high mortality (Table 20.1).

During treatment it is important to re-examine the patient frequently and consider:

- Persistent tachycardia – consider more fluid
- Cold peripheries and increased capillary refill time aim for <3°C core-peripheral difference and less than 3 s respectively
- Tachypnoea/hypoxia

Table 20.1 Glasgow Meningococcal Septicaemia Prognostic Score

BP <75 mmHg systolic, age <4 years; <85 mmHg systolic, >4 years	3
Skin/rectal temperature difference >3°C	3
Modified coma scale score <8 or deterioration of >3 points in 1 h	3
Deterioration in perceived clinical condition in the hour before scoring	2
Absence of meningism	2
Extending purpuric rash or widespread ecchymoses	1
Base deficit (capillary or arterial) >−8	1
Total	15

- Confusion
- Hypotension – need to keep BP sufficient to maintain urine output above 1 ml/kg/h

Initial management
- Optimise oxygenation
- If poor respiratory effort or comatose will need early intubation and ventilation (but see below)
- Obtain IV/IO access. Take bloods for:

Blood cultures	– for diagnosis
FBC	– may see diplococci, low platelets
Clotting	– may be prolonged – DIC
U&E	– hypokalaemia/hyperkalaemia
	– poor renal function
Calcium	– low in severe disease
Magnesium	– low in severe disease
Glucose	– may be low
Acid-base status	– metabolic acidosis

- Give antibiotic either cefotaxime 50 mg/kg qds or ceftriaxone 80 mg/kg od
- Fluids   20 ml/kg 0.9% NaCl, 4.5% human albumin solution (HAS) or synthetic colloid

    repeat as necessary 20 ml/kg
- Inotropes consider after 40–60 ml/kg of fluid

    dobutamine initially at 10 mcg/kg/min

    dilute solution can be given peripherally
- Lumbar puncture should not be performed in a suspected meningo-coccal septicaemia because of risk of coning due to raised intra-cranial pressure

Elective ventilation
Advantages
- Reduces work of breathing, reduces myocardial oxygen require-ments and reduces risk of pulmonary oedema developing while high volume fluid replacement continues.
- Most children with a GMSPS of >8 will require ventilation because of cardiovascular instability or decreasing level of consciousness.
- However, induction with thiopentone can cause severe hypotension at conventional dosage by vasodilatation and reduced cardiac output. If possible commence inotropes before ventilation. Ketamine 1–2 mg/kg IV is more cardiovascularly stable and can be used but care with raised ICP.
- PEEP should be added to reduce pulmonary oedema; start at 5 cm H_2O.

INFECTION AND RELATED ILLNESS

20

Disadvantages
- May worsen cardiovascular status because of:
  - raised intra-thoracic pressure due to ventilation reducing venous return
  - sedation reducing endogenous catecholamines, in addition to effects of sedatives on cardiovascular system

Essential monitoring
- Central line – aim for CVP 12–14 cm H_2O
- Arterial line – blood pressure and gas monitoring
- Urinary catheter – urine output, i.e. adequate BP and circulatory volume
- Swan-Ganz catheter may help guide effectiveness of inotropes and fluid replacement
- In smaller children repeat echocardiography/trans-oesophageal doppler can give some indication of cardiac output trends with inotrope changes

Further treatment
Continued fluid replacement is the mainstay of treatment:
- Colloid: Use boluses of 10 ml/kg 4.5% HAS to keep CVP within above limits.

  Some children may require several times their circulating volume. The commonest mistake is to give too little fluid.

  Continual reassessment of capillary refill time, heart rate and core-peripheral temperature gradient is important. Consider colloid infusion of 1–3 ml/kg/h if frequent boluses are required.

  Crystalloid: Restrict crystalloids to two thirds of maintenance. This minimises leak of fluid from intra-vascular space into interstitial compartment. Use 10% dextrose/0.45% saline. Dextrose concentration may need to be increased if BM remains <5 mmol/l.

  Blood and blood products should be given as dictated by repeat haemoglobin, platelet and clotting levels.
- Inotropes

  Not an alternative to adequate fluid replacement. Start immediately if elective ventilation considered or if 40 ml/kg colloid required for resuscitation. Double doses every 5 min if no response.

  Note all inotropes work more effectively at normal blood pH. Therefore correction of this may help their effectiveness.
- Use dobutamine initially up to 20 μg/kg/min. If not sufficient commence adrenaline for 'cold' shock. May also need noradrenaline if the patient develops 'warm' shock.

Other therapies
Prostacyclin
The vasodilator, prostacyclin, has been used as a peripheral vasodilator for impending peripheral gangrene. It may also help reduce the

metabolic acidosis due to increased peripheral perfusion. It will counteract some of the peripheral effects of adrenaline. Dosage is 5–20 ng/kg/min via a separate central line lumen. There is no direct evidence that it is of benefit.

Bacterial anti-toxin
Recent studies on bacterial anti-toxin drugs has shown some benefit. However, the benefit is probably reduced by late administration of the drug.

Calcium
- Hypocalcaemia is an indicator of severe disease
- Bolus 0.2 ml/kg 10% calcium gluconate
- Consider infusion. Useful inotrope in neonates and infants.
- Needs separate central line lumen
- Monitor levels 6–8 hourly
- Recent evidence suggests that giving calcium may worsen mortality in animal models and that it should only be used in refractory hypotension

Hypomagnesaemia
If <0.75 mmol/l give 0.2 ml/kg of 50% MgSO$_4$ over 30 min. Care with hypotension during administration.
- Hypo or hyperkalaemia can occur
- Hypoglycaemia
- Frequent BM monitoring and increase dextrose in fluids as necessary

Steroids
- Dexamethasone 0.4 mg/kg bd for 2 days (if meningitis present) is sometimes given but not recommended
- Hydrocortisone 1 mg/kg/dose tds for up to 5 days. May be useful to help catecholamine dependence. Measure cortisol first.

DIC
- Treat if clinical signs of bleeding. Prolongation of prothrombin time is an indicator of severity of disease.
- Discuss with haematologist recorrection with FFP/cryoprecipitate/platelets
- Also consider Vitamin K

Protein C
- Evidence that aggressive correction of the disturbance of coagulation modulators (protein C, protein S, antithrombin III) improves outcome

20

- Reduced mortality in critically ill adults using activated Protein C
- Measured levels of Protein C in meningococcal disease are often less than 10% of normal
- Rate of serious bleeding double that of controls

Metabolic acidosis
- Correct with sodium bicarbonate
- May respond to fluids and/or prostacyclin

Other possible problems
- Raised ICP
- Seizures
- Poor urine output – consider CVVH
- Plastic surgical referral for ischaemic limbs. Consider compartment pressure measurement and possible escharotomies.

Other diagnostic requirements
- Throat swab
- Skin scrapings
- Rapid antigen screen
- PCR
- Convalescent serology
- Convalescent CSF

Prophylaxis
- Rifampicin or ciprofloxacillin to child and contacts (close family)
- Consider staff prophylaxis only if in close proximity to patient's fluids
- Vaccination if appropriate strain identified

Human immunodeficiency virus infection
- Usually transmitted by vertical transmission from mother. This can be reduced by anti-retroviral therapy in pregnancy.
- Length of illness is shorter than in adults
- Many have protected asymptomatic phase
- Diagnosis can be made by PCR
- Admission to PICU usually due to respiratory failure (Table 20.2)

Pneumocystis carinii pneumonia (PCP)
- Commonly occurs in patients with AIDS particularly in first year of life
- Presents with cough, fever, tachypnoea and dyspnoea
- Signs include respiratory distress as there is ventilation-perfusion mismatch, reduced pulmonary compliance. Hypoxia may or may not be present.

Table 20.2 Respiratory causes of admission to PICU with AIDS

Bacterial	*Steptococcus pneumoniae, Haemophilus influenzae, Staphylococcus aureus* Nosocomial: *Pseudomonas aeruginosa* Mycobacterial: *Mycobacterium tuberculosis*
Viral	RSV, herpes simplex, varicella zoster, influenzae, parainfluenzae, adenovirus, measles, CMV
Fungal	Candida, aspergillus
Parasite	*Pneumocystis carinii*, toxoplasma
Non-infectious	Lymphoid disease Bronchiectasis Kaposi's sarcoma

Diagnosis
- Pulmonary secretions usually from broncho-pulmonary lavage can result in organism
- Open lung biopsy usually has 97% success rate of identifying the organism
- Chest X-ray usually shows diffuse interstitial infiltrates
- An isolated raised serum lactate dehydrogenase level
- CD4 count is often low

Treatment
- High dose co-trimoxazole initially intra-venously
- High dose corticosteroids are also effective but must be sure that CMV or miliary tuberculosis do not coexist as these may worsen
- Ventilate with high PEEP and pressure-limited to reduce lung damage, allowing permissive hypercapnia
- High frequency oscillation and surfactant have helped
- Mortality has reduced to 50–60%
- But prophylaxis is still indicated

Viral pneumonia
- This can occur as either a respiratory infection, e.g. RSV or as part of a disseminated viral infection, e.g. measles, CMV
- CMV pneumonitis can mimic PCP but tends to have a more insidious onset and is often not diagnosed until post mortem or lung biopsy
- Bronchoalveolar lavage may demonstrate CMV present due to viral shedding
- Ganciclovir 5 mg/kg bd is often used. Side effects include bone marrow depression, GI haemorrhage, nephrotoxicity.
- Steroids may worsen the CMV infection in children with AIDS
- Ribavirin can be used for patients with RSV infection

Mycobacterial pneumonia
- Signs and symptoms include fever, weight loss, cough, hilar lymphadenopathy, pulmonary infiltrates and consolidation
- Can be due to *Mycobacterium tuberculosis* or *M.avium-intracellulare*
- Testing by Mantoux testing
- Treatment should include isoniazid, rifampacin, pyrazinamide, streptomycin

Lymphoid diseases
- Occurs in 25–50% of perinatally acquired HIV
- Restrictive lung disease with hypoxia and hypocapnia
- Symptoms include cough, tachypnoea, wheezing, lymphadenopathy, hepatosplenomegaly, parotid enlargement
- Chest X-ray shows reticulonodular pattern and mediastinal lymph-adenopathy
- May need lung biopsy for diagnosis
- Treatment is supportive and may need long-term oxygen
- Upper airway obstruction can occur due to infectious causes, e.g. larygnotracheobronchitis. Laryngoscopy or bronchoscopy may be helpful.

Cardiovascular complications
- Arrhythmias
- Congestive cardiac failure
- Dilated cardiomyopathy
- Endocarditis
- Diagnosis usually by echocardiography
- Treatment is symptomatic

Renal complications
- Acute renal failure due to complications of septic shock or due to toxic effects of drug therapy
- HIV nephropathy with severe proteinuria. A glumerculosclerosis occurs. May be associated with renal tubular acidosis.
- Other parenchymal lesions such as interstitial nephritis or haemolytic-uraemic syndrome can occur
- Treatment may involve use of dialysis and management of fluid overload

Gastrointestinal complications
- Malnutrition with poor absorption and diarrhoea
- Pancreatitis
- Abnormal hepatic function
- Acute abdomen can occur

Table 20.3 Causes of neurological complications

HIV	• AIDS encephalopathy
	• Corticospinal tract degeneration
Opportunistic infection	• CMV encephalitis
	• Cerebral toxoplasmosis
	• Candida meningitis
	• Cryptococcal meningitis
Bacterial infection	• *Haemophilus influenzae* meningitis
	• *Streptococcal pneumonia* meningitis
Cerebral vascular accidents	

Neurological complications (Table 20.3)
- It is important to remember that these patients can have other causes for coma than those listed above.

Haematological complications
- Anaemia commonly due to chronic illness, poor nutrition and GI blood loss, and to drug toxicity
- Neutropenia is common at presentation
- Thrombocytopenia may lead to bleeding

Systemic inflammatory response syndrome (SIRS)

Septic episodes leading to bacteraemia may trigger various host responses causing the 'sepsis syndrome'. This process can also be caused by other events such as burns, trauma and reperfusion injury. The systemic inflammatory response is the final common pathway which may lead on to multi-system organ failure (MOSF) – (Table 20.4).

A suggested model for the various events that occur are:
- Bacteria have a lipopolysaccharide in their cell wall (endotoxin)
- This binds to receptors on monocytes and macrophages
- Cytokines are released – interleukin 1 (IL–1) and tumour necrosis factor (TNFα)
- These cytokines effect:
  - Temperature control – (fever, hypothermia)
  - Vascular resistance and permeability (hypotension, oedema)
  - Cardiovascular function (cardiac depression)
  - Bone marrow (increased WBC)
- Some end organ effects are mediated by nitric oxide, and arachidonic acid metabolites, e.g. prostaglandins, platelet activating factor
- Complex cytokine cascade is amplified and modified. IL-8 produced locally attracts neutrophils leading to local tissue damage and organ dysfunction.

INFECTION AND RELATED ILLNESS

20

Table 20.4 Clinical and pathophysiological manifestations of the continuum of SIRS

Stimulation (endotoxin, trauma, etc)
   Release of catecholamines
   Impaired cellular metabolism
   Transient peripheral vasodilation

Warm shock
   Continued cell injury
   Increased capillary permeability tends to reduced intra-vascular volume
   Increased cardiac output with peripheral vasodilation
   Decreased tissue perfusion

Cold shock
   Hypoxia
   Hypovolaemia and hypotension
   Vasoconstriction with cold peripheries
   Metabolic acidosis with increased lactate

Multi-system organ dysfunction/failure
   Heart failure
   Renal failure
   ARDS
   DIC
   Coma
   Irreversible ischaemia
   Death

- Complement, coagulation and kinin cascades are also stimulated
- Some anti-inflammatory products are also produced which try to modify this process
- Antibiotics although essential may exacerbate this process leading to more release of endotoxin

Treatment
- Antibiotics
- Surgery if this would eliminate source of infection
- Improvement of oxygen delivery
- Elimination of endotoxin (antisera)
- Mediator antagonism
- Anti-inflammatory drugs

CHAPTER 21

TRAUMA

Acute head injury

Head injury is the commonest cause of death in childhood over the age of 1. Approximately 40% of mortality in this age group involves head injury and there is considerable long-term morbidity.

History

Details of the injury can be obtained from parents, paramedics or witnesses once the child has been assessed fully and stabilised. Important features include:

- Length of unconsciousness
- Any evidence of seizures
- Any antecedent illness
- Is there a possibility of non-accidental injury?
  - Unconscious/encephalopathic without a cause
  - History does not explain the extent of injury
  - Bruises/other injuries not consistent with history

Examination

- Check and maintain airway – administer high flow oxygen.
- Stabilise cervical spine with hard neck collar.
- Cervical spine injury may be missed with potentially disastrous results until the patient is able to communicate that he or she has neck pain.
- Intubation in a head injured patient without adequate sedation may result in an increase in intra-cranial pressure. General anaesthesia with thiopentone as an induction agent helps attenuate this. The child should also be administered a muscle relaxant for the intubation in order to rapidly obtain airway protection (Table 21.1).
- Oral intubation is always first line until CT scan of the head is performed.

Table 21.1 Indications for early intubation and ventilation

- GCS of 8 and or deteriorating
- Loss of gag/laryngeal reflexes
- Hypoxia/hypercarbia
  - PaO_2 <8 kPa or oxygen saturation <95%
  - $PaCO_2$ >6 kPa
- If the patient is hyperventilating and $PaCO_2$ <3.5 kPa
- Cheyne-Stokes breathing
- Other trauma requiring intubation and ventilation, e.g. chest injury

TRAUMA

21

- Avoid nasal intubation in basal skull fracture because of the risk of ascending infection into the cranial cavity.
- Features of basal skull fracture include:
  - periorbital haemorrhage
  - bruising behind the ears
  - blood or CSF otorrhoea or rhinorrhoea
- Maintenance of circulation is also vital as hypotension in patients with a head injury is associated with poor outcome due to reduction of cerebral perfusion pressure and the potential of secondary hypoxic injury to the brain.
- It is also important to exclude other major extracranial injury.

Neurological examination
Initial examination of the neurological system is by using AVPU, posture and the response of the pupils to light (Table 21.2). 'P' corresponds to a Glasgow Coma Scale of 8 (Table 21.3).

Table 21.2 The AVPU scale

A – Alert
V – Responds to voice
P – Responds to pain
U – Unresponsive
Pupils
Posture

Table 21.3 Glasgow Coma Scale

	Over 5 years old		Infants under 5	
Eye opening	Spontaneous	4	Spontaneous	4
	To voice	3	To speech	3
	To pain	2	To pain	2
	None	1	None	1
Verbal	Orientated	5	Coos and babbles	5
	Confused speech	4	Irritable cries	4
	Inappropriate words	3	Cries to pain	3
	Incomprehensible sounds	2	Moans to pain	2
	None	1	None	1
Motor	Obeys commands	6	Normal spontaneous movements	6
	Localises pain	5	Withdraws to touch	5
	Withdraws	4	Withdraws to pain	4
	Abnormal flexion	3	Abnormal flexion	3
	Extension	2	Abnormal extension	2
	None	1	None	1

More detailed neurological examination uses the Glasgow Coma Scale. This requires modification below the age of 5.

- Check GCS every 15 min for the first hour then half hourly to evaluate progress
- Check pupil size, equality and reaction to light. Dilated pupils may indicate raised intra-cranial pressure and a unilateral dilated pupil may suggest an extra-dural or sub-dural haemorrhage.
- Focal signs
- Fundoscopy – haemorrhage may be observed
- Eye movement
- Corneal and gag reflex
- Assess posture and tone

Indication of raised ICP
- Decreased level of consciousness
- Cushing's triad – hypertension, bradycardia and apnoea
- Persistent vomiting
- Squint, III or VI nerve palsy
- Unequal or dilated pupils
- Papilloedema is rare in acute head injury
- In infants, a full fontanelle or sutural separation may be present
- Retinal or vitreous haemorrhage – associated with poor outcome

Indications for cranial CT scan
Nearly all children will need elective intubation and ventilation for the scan.
- GCS less than 12 or deteriorating
- Presence of focal neurological signs
- Persistent seizures
- Other signs of raised ICP
- Infant with unexplained encephalopathic illness or if non-accidental injury (NAI) suspected
- Consider CT or ultrasound abdomen at same time if multiple trauma to assess the possibility of intra-abdominal injury

CT scan criteria for raised ICP
- Effacement of the basal cisterns
- Thin slit-like ventricles or completely obliterated
- Cortical sulci obliterated
- Shift in the midline, herniation of temporal lobe or cerebellar tonsils

TRAUMA

21

- If CT shows any signs of extra-dural or sub-dural haemorrhage needs immediate discussion with and transfer to neurosurgical centre for possible surgery
- if in need of ventilation discuss with PICU

Indications for admission to PICU
- GCS of less than 10 or deteriorating
- Presence of focal neurological signs
- Persistent seizures
- Multiple trauma
- All intubated children

Indications for ICP monitoring
- GCS 8 or less
- Abnormal CT scan – tight brain
- Post neurosurgery
- Some patients with meningitis, encephalitis and metabolic encephalopathy may benefit from ICP monitoring
- Hypertension and abnormal posturing

May not be appropriate if patient has GCS of 3 with fixed dilated pupils.

Methods of ICP monitoring
- Intra-ventricular catheter
  - Gold standard placed in lateral ventricle
  - Measures direct pressure from the CSF in the ventricles
  - Accurate
  - Can be used therapeutically to remove CSF
  - May be difficult to insert
  - Risk of infection and intra-cranial bleeding
- Fibreoptic transducer
  - Reasonably accurate
  - Can be intra-parenchymal, epidural or sub-arachnoid
  - Tip of catheter is reference point therefore does not need frequent calibration
  - Easy to insert
- Epidural or sub-arachnoid catheters
  - Problems with accuracy and drift leading to a tendency to over-read
  - Easy to insert

Indications for jugular venous bulb monitoring
- Technique for measuring oxygen consumption of the brain leading to an assessment of the adequacy of global cerebral blood flow

- Fibreoptic probe passed retrograde from internal jugular vein to the jugular venous bulb at the base of the skull
- Normal saturations 65–70%
- Assumption has to be made about adequate delivery (haemoglobin, arterial oxygen saturation)
- Reduced levels suggest hypoperfusion, <40% implies ischaemia
- Rises suggest cerebral hyperaemia
- Cerebral lactate production can be measured
- Treatment of a falling level may indicate the need to raise CPP, FiO_2 or haemoglobin

Intra–cranial pressure

Cerebral perfusion pressure (CPP) = mean arterial pressure (MAP) − intra–cranial pressure (ICP)

Normal ICP is less than 15 mmHg.
Causes of raised ICP are given in Table 21.4.

Effects of raised ICP
- Signs of raised ICP include headache, vomiting and papilloedema
- Acute raised ICP may lead to tonsillar or transtentori herniation with signs of bradycardia, hypertension, irregular respiration and fixed and dilated pupils leading to death
- Variation in cerebral blood flow in the normal brain is autoregulated with variation in the cerebral perfusion pressure

Treatment
- The essentials are supportive until recovery:
  - Adequate oxygenation
  - Adequate blood flow to brain by maintaining CPP
  - Avoiding or treating fits promptly
  - Treat pain
  - Diagnose and treat intra–cranial bleeds

Table 21.4 Causes of raised intra-cranial pressure

• Mass:	blood – haemorrhage	
	tumour	
	abscess	
• Increased blood flow:	vasodilatation, e.g. injury, hypoxia, hypercarbia	
	venous obstruction	
	abnormal structure, e.g. arterio-venous malformation	
• Increased CSF:	hydrocephalus	
• Increased tissue:	oedema	injury
		around tumour
		metabolic or hepatic encephalopathy
	osmotic	following resuscitation, e.g. in diabetic ketoacidosis (DKA)

TRAUMA

21

Essentially treatment can be stratified depending on GCS, CT scan and ICP findings. Frequently children will be transferred and admitted to PICU following the need for anaesthesia for a CT scan for a child with a reduced GCS. Management depends on local policies but can be divided into:

- GCS 9 or above with a normal CT scan can be allowed to wake up and neurological assessment undertaken
- GCS 3 with fixed dilated pupils and an abnormal brain scan are probably brain dead and sedation is not required to enable early neurological assessment
- GCS 4–8 inclusive or those above GCS 9 with an abnormal brain scan, raised ICP or other injuries requiring ventilation should be sedated and ventilated until evidence of reduced cerebral oedema either sustained reduction in ICP or improvement on serial CT brain scans

Cerebral perfusion pressure is also affected by:

- Pain and anxiety
- Increased metabolic demand (increased temperature)
- Epileptic seizures

Principles of head injury management

- Keep CPP above 50 mmHg if possible
- Keep $PaCO_2$ low normal – 4.5 kPa. Lower $PaCO_2$ leads to reduced cerebral blood flow and may worsen cerebral ischaemia.
- Keep patient well sedated to avoid surges of ICP with suction, coughing, straining, physiotherapy
- Consider neuro-muscular paralysis if necessary
- Keep head straight to avoid kinking of jugular veins and head up 20–30° to help reduce venous pressure (hard neck-collar may increase venous pressure)
- Relative fluid restriction to reduce intra-cerebral water, but it is important to resuscitate the child properly
- Maintain CPP by increasing mean arterial pressure through adequate resuscitation fluid and inotropes if necessary, e.g. norepinephrine
- Make sure glucose levels are maintained at normal levels as high glucose causes neurological damage and is highly likely during the early stages following injury due to the stress response – use 0.9% saline until glucose is in the normal range
- Consider prophylactic anti-convulsants

Treatment of raised ICP

- Remove masses
- Hyperventilation has a temporary effect
- Osmotic diuretics – mannitol. This can however cross the blood-brain barrier and worsen cerebral oedema after the first few doses.

Maximum 1.5 g/kg in the first 24 h. A dose of 0.25–0.5 g/kg initially is indicated. Make sure the serum osmolality remains below 315 mOsm/l.

- 3% sodium chloride (5 ml/kg) is more physiological and tends to draw water out of the cerebral cells. Furosemide can also be used.

- Steroids are useful only in patients with cerebral masses particularly tumours

- Barbiturate induced coma can be considered

Other therapies
- Physiotherapy and particularly suction lead to an increase in ICP. Bolus sedation with, e.g. alfentanil is useful.

- Temperature increase leads to an increase in cerebral metabolic rate and blood flow. There is no evidence as yet that hypothermia is therapeutic but measures should be taken to avoid hyperthermia:
  - cooling (cooling blankets, ice)
  - paracetamol
  - NSAIDs, e.g. ibuprofen (if no problems with renal failure or clotting)
  - chlorpromazine IV (0.1 mg/kg slowly) – this is a very low dose and sometimes helps reduce pyrexia probably by acting centrally. However care with possible hypotension.

- Seizures are fairly common following acute head injury, the use of EEG or cerebral function monitoring is necessary particularly if the patient is paralysed. Phenytoin (18 mg/kg) loading dose may be used prophylactically.

- Consider urinary catheterisation, to monitor urine output and to prevent ICP rise due to a full bladder

- Surgery for extra-dural or sub-dural bleeds. Conservative treatment of small haemorrhages requires appropriate CT scanning if the patient deteriorates.

- Surgery can be used for bony injury, e.g. depressed skull fracture or for acute hydrocephalus

- Decompressive craniotomy may also be used. If it is used it probably needs to be used early and requires ICP monitoring to be instigated.

- Avoid hypo-osmolar state as this leads to increased cerebral oedema

Non–accidental injury

Can present in various ways which can be a problem with differential diagnosis. Needs to be considered in infants with unexplained altered level of consciousness.

- unexplained coma or fits
- unexplained trauma with healing fractures often of different ages or unusual or inconsistent with history

TRAUMA

21

- isolated burns, e.g. of buttocks, scalded hands and feet, cigarette burns
- unexplained bruising

Diagnosis
- suspicion
- clinical: full fontanelle, retinal haemorrhages
- ultrasound or CT of head looking for extradural or sub-dural haematomas, skull fractures
- skeletal survey

Treatment should be symptomatic for the presenting features. Involvement of appropriate paediatricians, social services and police is important for investigating the circumstances and protecting other siblings.

Thoracic trauma
- Blunt trauma commonest
- Often quite high potential transmission of energy due to elastic chest
- High incidence of pulmonary contusion
- Airway
  - Obstruction
  - Blood
  - Gastric contents
  - Direct trauma – disruption
- Breathing
  - Pneumothorax (simple, tension, open)
  - Diaphragmatic rupture
- Circulation
  - Tamponade
  - Disruption of great vessels

Treatment
- Airway and oxygen
- Needle thoracocentesis
- Chest drain insertion
- Fluid and blood replacement
- Pericardiocentesis
- Referral to cardiothoracic centre

Abdominal trauma
- Usually due to blunt trauma
- Injuries to liver and spleen due to less protection and larger size more common than in adults

- Injury to bowel, renal tract, massive peritoneal or retroperitoneal haemorrhage can also occur
- Treatment is usually conservative following radiological imaging CT or ultrasound
- Indications for laparotomy include:
  - hypovolaemia
  - persistent haemorrhage
  - gastrointestinal perforation
  - signs of peritonism
  - increased intra-abdominal pressure
  - non-functioning kidney

Spinal injury
- Difficulty of interpretation of X-rays. Better if lateral cervical X-ray and CT are available together. MRI gives better soft tissue views.
- Risk of spinal cord injury without obvious radiological abnormality (SCIWORA) leading to severe complications
- Keep a high index of suspicion and therefore keep cervical spine immobilised and log roll the patient with in-line stabilisation
- Lumbar spinal injuries can be caused by a lap seat belt
- Clinical examination and absence of pain in the neck with normal X-rays is the best way of ensuring clearance of the cervical spine
- However in the semi-conscious child in whom it is not clear whether the neck is clear, they may be difficult to restrain and then it is safer to let them move, keeping their neck as in-line as possible with a more comfortable collar

Drowning
- death is due to asphyxia usually within 24 h of insult
- near drowning is survival beyond 24 h
- recovery depends on degree of hypoxic insult
- may develop hypervolaemia due to fluid absorbtion via gastric and pulmonary circulations leading to fluid shift from the extra-cellular space
- hypovolaemia can occur due to fluid shifts into the third space
- care with full stomach – risk of vomiting and aspiration
- hyperglycaemia or hypoglycaemia can occur
- no difference between fresh and salt water drowning

Pulmonary effects
- during drowning event, hypoxia and hypercarbia develop rapidly leading to respiratory and then metabolic acidosis
- aspiration of fluid occurs leading to V/Q mismatch worsening hypoxia
- effect of water on surfactant leads to atelectasis and increased intra-pulmonary shunt

- secondary deterioration may be due to continuing loss of surfactant, pneumonia, barotrauma, ARDS, unrecognised foreign body aspiration

Cardiovascular effects
- usually develop cardiogenic shock:
    - with poor cardiac contractility
    - increased capillary permeability
    - increased systemic vascular resistance

Other effects
- these are essential due to the hypoxic insult to the body
- renal failure
- liver dysfunction
- GI dysfunction including possible perforation
- disseminated intra-vascular coagulation (DIC)
- often develop cerebral oedema 24–48 h post event
- trauma at time of drowning, e.g. head injury

Management
- low threshold for intubation and ventilation
- high concentration oxygen and positive end expiratory pressure (PEEP)

Cardiovascular
- arrhythmias common – bradycardia, asystole (warm water); atrial or ventricular fibrillation (cold water)
- if the patient presents in ventricular fibrillation (VF) try DC shocks but may remain in VF if hypothermic especially below 30°C
- maintain cardiac output with cardio-pulmonary resuscitation (CPR) until rewarmed
- care with fluid boluses

Hypothermia
Rewarming should include:
- surface   – heaters, warming blankets
- core   – humidified gases, warmed IV fluids, gastric, peritoneal or rectal lavage, cardio-pulmonary bypass
- should not be declared dead until core temperature above 32°C if possible
- may have increase in metabolic acidosis when peripheral perfusion improves

Predictive variables
- not completely diagnostic but poor outcome more likely if:
  - no heart rate on arrival at hospital
  - submersion more than 10 min in non-icy water with more than 25 min of CPR
  - need for cardiac drugs during resuscitation

better outcome is likely if:
- submersion of 5 min or less with less than 10 min of CPR
- sinus rhythm, reactive pupils and response at scene

Treatment
Aim to minimise cerebral damage by:
- rapid restoration of oxygenation and circulation
- correction of metabolic and electrolyte abnormalities
- maintenance of normal temperature and blood glucose
- control seizures
- control raised ICP

Therapies are aimed to keep ICP under control:
- sedate and paralyse
- avoid noxious stimuli causing raised ICP
- elevate head to 20–30°
- ventilate to $PaCO_2$ of about 4.5 kPa
- avoid fluid overload
- diuretics – mannitol/furosemide

Assessment of neurological function
- CT scan – abnormal within 36 h is associated with poor prognosis
- EEG – demonstrating signs compatible with hypoxic brain damage
- Clinical examination after cessation of sedatives

Burns
- serious burns requiring PICU are few <100 per year in the UK
- severe burns are defined as >15% surface area
  - or a full-thickness of greater 5%
  - or smoke inhalation
  - or carbon monoxide poisoning
- remember other possible trauma, e.g. in explosions

Initial care
- Assess airway
- Stop burning process
- Begin fluid resuscitation

TRAUMA

21

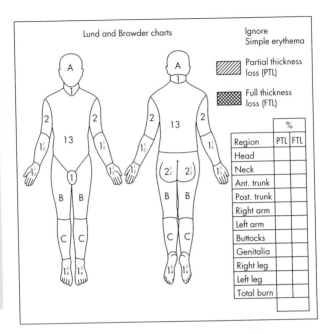

Figure 21.1 Lund and Browder charts.

Table 21.5 Surface area of head and legs with age (%)

	Age in years				
	0	1	5	10	15
A = half head	9.5	8.5	6.5	5.5	4.5
B = half thigh	2.75	3.25	4.0	4.5	4.5
C = half lower leg	2.5	2.5	2.75	3.0	3.25

Assessment of the burn

Surface area
- estimated using burn charts
- surface area of head and legs vary with age
- palm and adducted fingers form 1% of the body surface area
- the rule of nines does not apply until about 14 years of age

Assessment of the burn area is by use of the Lund + Browder chart (see Figure 21.1). The relative size of the head and legs varies with age and this is demonstrated in Table 21.5.

Table 21.6 Reasons for intubation in burns include

- CNS depression
- airway burns/facial burns
- inhalational injury
- pneumonia or sepsis
- surgery

Depth

- superficial burns are an injury to the epidermis causing redness but no blisters

- partial-thickness burns cause some damage to the dermis. The skin is usually pink or mottled with blisters. These areas are very painful.

- full-thickness burns damage both the epidermis and dermis and may cause injury to deeper structures. The skin appears white, charred and leathery and is usually painless.

- may need to give an elective general anaesthetic with rapid sequence induction (Table 21.6).

- if thermal injury to airway, oedema will develop quickly and early intubation may be life saving. May be a difficult intubation due to the airway oedema.

- care with use of suxamethonium. From 2 days after injury, cells are more likely to release potassium after suxamethonium is given leading to hyperkalaemia causing arrhythmias.

Fluid management

- patients require fluids for:
  - resuscitation
  - normal maintenance
  - burn area

- insert a central venous line to assess intra-vascular volume

- aim to keep good urine output – catheterise and keep flow of at least 0.5–1 ml/kg/h

- diuretics only necessary in some cases of soft tissue or electrical injury to help prevent myoglobin associated renal failure

- fluid required is
  - maintenance as crystalloid
  - colloid as crystalloid at 4 ml/kg/% burn
  - half in first 8 h from time of burn
  - rest in next 16 h

- reassess electrolytes, fluid status regularly

- additional boluses 20 ml/kg for resuscitation

- alternatively crystalloid can be used for resuscitation

TRAUMA

21

Blood tests
- FBC, U&E, cross-match
- arterial blood gas measurements for acid-base, carboxyhaemoglobin and cyanide levels

Analgesia
- adequate analgesia by opiate infusion
- check that distress is not due to hypoxia
- initial wound care with cling film
- check limbs for circumferential burns and the need for surgical escharotomies

General principles of ICU management of burns
- sterility to avoid infections
- appropriate surgical intervention with skin grafting, the earlier the better
- nutrition – enteral route preferred
  - early commencement ideally within 4 h
  - increase in calories given, dependent on surface area of burn
- psychological aspects of burn to patient and family need addressing

Smoke inhalation
- causes considerable number of deaths by:
  - causing thermal injury
  - carbon monoxide poisoning
  - cyanide poisoning
  - pulmonary injury
  - hypoxia
- hypoxia worsens mental function and ability to escape fire

Carbon monoxide
- carbon monoxide is rapidly taken up in the lungs of children to combine with haemoglobin to form carboxyhaemoglobin
- carboxyhaemoglobin needs to be measured but smoke inhalation cannot be ruled out even if the level is normal
- normal pulse oximeter readings can occur due to absorption of light by carboxyhaemoglobin although the content of oxygen in the blood is reduced
- causes many different effects on organ systems including arrhythmias, pulmonary oedema
- classically, as the percentage of carbon monoxide increases there is:
  - increasing shortness of breath
  - increasing headache and fatigue

- increasing confusion leading to coma and death
- cutaneous dilatation

Treatment
- Oxygen reduces the half life of carbon monoxide from 5 to 6 h in air to one and a half hours in 100%
- Hyperbaric oxygen should be considered as this speeds up this process
- Intubation and ventilation if appropriate
- Severe acidosis is generally a poor prognostic sign

Cyanide poisoning
- usually combined with carbon monoxide poisoning
- difficult to measure levels rapidly
- signs include headache, dizziness, nausea and vomiting, tachypnoea leading to shock, coma and respiratory arrest

Treatment with amylnitrite inhalation (0.3 ml); 3% sodium nitrite 0.2–0.4 ml/kg IV over 3 min and sodium thiosulphate 25% solution 1.6 ml/kg IV over 10 min.

Lung injury
- mucosal oedema and sloughing
- increased lung permeability
- increased lung water
- ciliary function decreased
- altered surfactant production

Clinical features
- bronchospasm
- atelectasis and consolidation leading to pneumonia
- pulmonary oedema

Treatment
- oxygen
- ventilation
- pulmonary toilet to remove soot and plugs of secretions
- antibiotics for infection, often Staphylococcus early, Pseudomonas later

Electrocution
- deep burn through tissues
- entry and exit wounds
- cardiac arrest common
- ventricular fibrillation precipitated by current through heart
- primary respiratory arrest or asphyxiation due to chest wall tetany

TRAUMA

21

- loss of consciousness or seizures
- acute renal failure due to myoglobin or direct electrical injury
- haemorrhage and thrombosis

Treatment
- cardio-pulmonary resuscitation
- fluid to maintain good urine output, often requiring more than expected for the surface burn area
- fasciotomy of damaged area

CHAPTER 22

POISONING

- Accidental ingestion in children account for 80–90% of admissions
- In teenagers, suicide attempts or overdose of recreational drugs is more likely
- Table 22.1 lists the commonest agents ingested

History
- consider poisoning in any unexplained illness of sudden onset
- evidence of taking – observed, empty bottles
- maximum dose
- time since dose
- route of administration
- history before presentation to hospital
- family drug history
- symptoms may fall into a toxidrome (Table 22.2)

Management
- Mainly supportive as appropriate (ABC)
  - intubate and ventilate
  - fluids
  - monitoring

Table 22.1 Common causative agents of poisoning in children (from Woolf A et al. Poisoning and the critically ill child. In: Rogers MC and Helfaer MA. Handbook of Pediatric Intensive Care 3rd edn. Williams and Wilkins, Baltimore, 1999)

Anti-arrhythmics	Alcohol
Anti-convulsants	Ethylene glycol
Anti-histamines	Caustics
Anti-hypertensives	Glue
Aminophylline	Herbicides
Aspirin	Organophosphates
β blockers	Pesticides
Calcium channel blockers	Petroleum
Digoxin	
Hallucinogens	
Iron	
Opioids	
Oral hypoglycaemic agents	
Paracetamol	
Tricyclic anti-depressants	

22

Table 22.2 Toxidromes (from Mofenson HC, Greensher J. The unknown poison. Reproduced with permission from Pediatrics, Vol 54, 336–42,1974)

Drug involved	Clinical manifestations
Anti-cholinergics (atropine, scopolamine, tricyclic anti-depressants, phenothiazines, anti-histamines, mushrooms)	Agitation, hallucinations, coma, extrapyramidal movements, mydriasis, flushed, warm dry skin, dry mouth, tachycardia, arrhythmias, hypotension, hypertension, decreased bowel sounds, urinary retention
Cholinergics (organophosphates and carbamate insecticides)	Salivation, lacrimation, urination, defaecation, nausea, and vomiting, sweating, miosis, bronchorrhea, rales and wheezes, weakness, paralysis, confusion and coma, muscle fasciculations
Opiates	Slow respiration, bradycardia, hypotension, hypothermia, coma, miosis, pulmonary oedema, seizures
Sedative/hypnotics	Coma, hypothermia, central nervous system depression, slow respiration, hypotension, tachycardia
Tricyclic anti-depressants	Coma, convulsions, arrhythmias, anti-cholinergic manifestations
Salicylates	Vomiting, hyperpnoea, fever, lethargy, coma
Phenothiazines	Hypotension, tachycardia, torsion of head and neck, oculogyric crisis, trismus, ataxia, anti-cholinergic manifestations
Sympathomimetics (amphetamines, phenylpropanolamine, ephedrine, caffeine, cocaine, and aminophylline)	Tachycardia, arrhythmias, psychosis, hallucinations, delirium, nausea, vomiting, abdominal pain, piloerection
Alcohols, Glycols (methanol, ethylene glycol) also Salicylates, Paraldehyde, Iron, Isoniazid, Phenformin	Elevated anion gap metabolic acidosis

Reduce exposure

Methods depend on:

- patient's age
- substances ingested
- time since ingestion

• there is no place for emetics in children

• gastric lavage

- often needs general anaesthetic to protect airway
- useful for recent ingestion
- avoid if corrosive substances ingested

- activated charcoal may be useful up to 24 h after ingestion particularly if slow release preparations taken or if drugs which are slowly absorbed have been ingested. Repeated doses may help reduce absorption in drugs which have entero-hepatic circulation.
- cathartics – reduce absorption by decreasing transit time
- whole bowel irrigation by isotonic polyethylene glycol electrolyte solutions can be used for drugs not absorbed by activated charcoal but have a long transit time (e.g. iron) treatment at 30 ml/kg/h should continue until the diarrhoea induced becomes clear fluid
- surgery, e.g. to remove cocaine/morphine packets

Increase elimination
- diuresis with or without alkalisation by sodium bicarbonate is used for salicylate poisoning and other weak acids. Maintain a pH >6.0.
- haemodialysis – most useful for small molecular weight drugs with a small volume of distribution and poor protein binding, e.g. salicylates, lithium
- charcoal haemoperfusion can absorb polar and non-polar drugs such as barbiturates and digoxin
- haemofiltration can help remove large compounds, e.g. aminoglycoside or theophylline. It can also be useful with iron or lithium.
- exchange transfusion may be useful if methaemoglobinaemia has been caused

Investigations
- routine bloods including electrolytes
- paracetamol and salicylate levels will give an indication of amounts taken and help with treatment options
- gastric washouts should be sent for analysis
- urine toxicology should be analysed

Corrosive liquid ingestion
- alkalis tend to cause more damage than acids
- liquids cause more scars than solids
- batteries or other solids stuck in the oesophagus cause most damage
- treatment is symptomatic
- neutralisation not recommended
- no evidence of steroids being useful
- long-term scarring may occur

Specific treatments
- Benzodiazepines   – flumazenil
- Opiates   – naloxone

POISONING

22

- Paracetamol
  - N-acetylcysteine
  - may be useful beyond first 24 h
  - monitoring of prothrombin time and liver function tests necessary
- Iron
  - desferrioxamine
  - whole bowel irrigation
- Tricyclic anti-depressants
  - monitoring for arrhythmias
  - sodium bicarbonate 8.4% 1 ml/kg bolus repeated to keep pH 7.45–7.55
  - activated charcoal may help reduce absorption

Recreational drugs

Cocaine
- cocaine overdose leads to hallucinations, agitation, convulsions, hypertension, myocardial ischaemia, cerebral infarction and particularly cardiac arrhythmias
- use activated charcoal if ingestion within 1 h
- benzodiazepines are useful for agitation and convulsions
- calcium antagonists may be useful for resistant arrhythmias
- treat acidosis as this exacerbates arrhythmias

Ecstasy
- amphetamine derivative producing euphoria, stimulation and mood alteration
- produces idiosynchratic reactions including coma, convulsions, arrhythmias, malignant hyperthermia, rhabdomyolysis, hypertension and multi-organ failure; can mimic febrile convulsions
- activated charcoal may be useful if within 1 h of ingestion
- blood levels can be measured to determine consumption
- signs of cardiac or neurological toxicity require intensive care and monitoring
- hyperthermia may respond to cooling measures or require dantrolene 1 mg/kg over 10–15 min repeated up to a maximum of 10 mg/kg in 24 h
- labetalol can be used for hypertension and benzodiazepines for sedation
- fluid management can be problematical. Water intoxication can have occurred at presentation, but the patient may be dehydrated and a diuresis may be required to clear myoglobin.

LSD – lysergic acid diethylamide
- 5-HT agonist causing hallucination
- rapid absorption and duration of action

POISONING

- symptomatic treatment is indicated as required, avoid pheno-thiazides

Further information
Drug toxicity information is available at:
National Poisons Information Service
TOXBASE on the internet at www.spib.axl.co.uk/toxbase/
National telephone number at 0870 600 6266

CHAPTER 23

NEONATAL AND OTHER SURGICAL PATIENTS IN PICU

In addition to the problems of neonates and post-operative major surgery the following conditions have specific potential problems.

Congenital diaphragmatic hernia
- incidence of 1 in 4000 live births
- problem is reduction of lung tissue with abdominal contents within the thoracic cavity. A nasogastric tube may reduce ventilation compromise.
- poorly formed diaphragm usually on left. Associated with malrotation of the gut. 25% have associated cardiovascular anomalies.
- main problem is persistent pulmonary hypertension
- repair is not urgent
- needs to be stable for 24 h pre-operatively
- mortality 40–50% of live births which has not changed significantly over the last 30 years
- hypoxia may be persistent

Ventilation
- conventional ventilation needs to be fast (60 bpm) with small tidal volume. High frequency oscillation is probably more advantageous.
- may not be able to reduce $PaCO_2$ to normal
- weaning may be prolonged

Tracheo-oesophageal fistula
- occurs approximately in 1 out of 4500 live births
- associated with other anomalies
- major problem pre-operatively is ventilation through the fistula leading to distension of the stomach, splinting of the diaphragm and reduction in effective ventilation
- post-operatively may need ventilating to allow healing of the surgical anastomosis of the oesophagus. Some surgeons like about 5 days for a tight repair.
- H-type fistulas may be a cause of recurrent chest infections in infancy

Gastroschisis/exomphalus
- problem is the compression of abdominal contents back into the small abdomen, creating diaphragmatic splinting and requiring post-operative ventilation

- may need to replace the abdominal contents over some days using gortex patch to protect the bowel
- risk of moderate to large losses of serous fluid
- risk of temperature loss

Spinal surgery
Patients undergoing spinal surgery have a number of potential problems:
- restrictive lung defect leading to requirement for ventilation post-operatively
- poor cough
- other major neurological or neuro-muscular co-morbidity
- major surgery requiring:
  - post-operative analgesia
  - major peri-operative blood loss
  - potential neurological damage to spinal cord
- monitoring of neurological function in the legs is required
- care with blood loss especially on release of the clamps of the drainage bottles

Neurosurgery
- commonly post trauma, tumour surgery
- principles when ventilated are:
  - to maintain low normal $PaCO_2$ (c. 4.5 kPa)
  - keep head up tilt moderately at 10–20°
  - keep head straight to avoid increased venous pressure from kinked jugular veins
  - avoid fall in cerebral perfusion pressure by preventing ICP rise and hypotension
  - good sedation and analgesia
  - avoid physiotherapy and suction as much as possible
- particular problems after posterior fossa surgery include:
  - loss of gag reflex leading to possibility of aspiration
  - neurogenic pulmonary oedema
  - cerebral haemorrhage
  - hydrocephalus
  - consider problems with analgesia especially the effect of morphine on conscious level
- need for steroids
- increased incidence of epilepsy

23

Section 3

Drugs Used in Paediatric Intensive Care

DRUGS USED IN PAEDIATRIC INTENSIVE CARE

Aciclovir
A purine nucleoside analogue

Use
- Anti-viral agent for treatment of Herpes infections

Dose
<3 months   10 mg/kg tds
3 months–12 years   250 mg/m^2 tds
>12 years   12 mg/kg tds
Double dose in severe infections over 3 months
Reduce dose frequency in renal failure

Side effects
Phlebitis and local inflammation at site of injection
Polyuric renal failure (reversible)
Increased risk of renal failure with other nephrotoxic drugs
CNS toxicity (tremors, confusion and fits)

Adenosine
Endogenous nucleoside which slows atrioventricular (AV) node conduction and prolongs PR interval

Uses
- Supraventricular tachycardia termination (not atrial flutter or AF)
- Diagnosis of a broad complex tachycardia

Dose
50 μg/kg IV rapidly with flush
Increase in increments of 50 μg/kg every 2 min
Max   300 μg/kg <1 month
        500 μg/kg >1 month

Contra-indications/warnings
2nd or 3rd degree heart block, sick sinus syndrome
Atrial flutter or fibrillation

Side effects
Flushing, dyspnoea, chest pain, bronchospasm

Alfentanil
Short acting opioid 5–10 min

Use
- Analgesia particularly for short procedures or as adjunct

Dose
5–50 µg/kg bolus
0.5–1 µg/kg/min infusion

Side effects
Respiratory depression if not ventilated
Transient fall in blood pressure and heart rate after administration
Nausea and vomiting
Increased length of action in hepatic failure

Aminophylline
Theophylline salt

Uses
- Bronchodilator
- Respiratory stimulant in babies with apnoeas
- Diuretic, useful with severe respiratory distress

Dose
Bronchodilator:
Loading dose   5 mg/kg IV over 20–30 min
                  250–500 mg over 12 years
                  Omit if on theophylline preparations
Infusion   1 mg/kg/h or 0.5 mg/kg/h over 12 years
Diuretic: 2–4 mg/kg synergistic effect if given 30 min before furosemide can be given as IV infusion

Contra-indications
Omit loading dose if on oral theophylline
Clearance reduces with reduced cardiac or hepatic function
Increased levels with cimetidine, erythromycin, ciprofloxacin
Decreased levels with rifampicin, carbamazepine, phenobarbitone, phenytoin
Increased risk of hypokalaemia with salbutamol

Side effects
Tachycardia, arrhythmias, convulsions, headache, decreased gastric emptying with increased risk of vomiting and reflux, hyperglycaemia
Monitor levels 10–20 mg/l (55–110 mmol/l)

Amiodarone
Anti-arrhythmic which prolongs the action potential in atrium and
ventricle

Use
- Ventricular and supraventricular arrhythmias. Causes little myocardial
  depression.

Dose
5 mg/kg po/IV max 200 mg. Initially given bd for 7–10 days as loading dose then od for maintenance.

Contra-indications/warnings
Thyroid dysfunction (contains iodine)
Sinus bradycardia or heart block
Circulatory collapse
Interactions with β blockers and calcium channel antagonists
Potentiates digoxin, warfarin, theophylline, phenytoin

Side effects – acute
Anaphylactic shock (rapid IV boluses)
Skin reactions
Nightmares
Corneal deposits (reversible) requires monitoring

Long-term
Pulmonary fibrosis, pneumonitis, alveolitis (reversible)
Raised liver function tests
Hypo or hyperthyroidism
Peripheral neuropathy, myopathy and cerebellar dysfunction (reversible)
Hepatitis leading to cirrhosis (rare)

Amitriptyline
Tricyclic anti-depressant with sedative properties

Use
- Depression, neuralgic pain

Dose
25 mg bd/tds or 75 mg nocte max 150 mg over 12 years old
Start low and titrate
Takes some time to reach therapeutic levels

Side effects
Sedation

Anti-cholinergic, e.g. dry mouth, cardiac dysrhythmias, sweating

Hyponatraemia

Interactions
Plasma concentration reduced by some anti-convulsants

Increased by phenothiazines, cimetidine

Amoxycillin
Broad spectrum penicillin

Uses
- active against gram-positive and some gram-negative bacteria
- inactivated by β-lactamases

Dose
30 mg/kg IV tds (dose may be doubled in severe infection)

50 mg/kg IV bd–qds in neonates depending on age

Maximum dose 4 g daily

Contra-indications/warnings
Allergy

Renal failure reduce frequency of administration

Prolongs prothrombin time with warfarin

Removed by haemodialysis/peritoneal dialysis

Side effects
Gastrointestinal – nausea, diarrhoea

Urtical or maculo-papular rash especially with glandular fever

Amphotericin
Polyene antifungal

Use
- Fungal infections including candida and aspergillus

Dose
Test dose recommended

Conventional   250 μg/kg increasing by 250 μg/kg/day to
                1 mg/kg od IV
                250 μg/kg for neonates

Liposomal   1 mg/kg increasing by 1 mg/kg/day to
                3 mg/kg od IV for all children
                5 mg/kg od for proven systemic infection

Contra-indications/warnings

Hypersensitivity

Renal impairment – reduce dose or stop if serum creatinine twice normal

Low serum potassium, magnesium and phosphate can occur

Side effects
- Acute infusion reactions such as fever, nausea, vomiting, headache, muscle and joint pains. Usually most severe and frequent with first dose. Thus use of test dose which can be covered by hydrocortisone.
- Nephrotoxicity occurs in >85% with abnormal electrolytes including hypokalaemia and raised urea and creatinine. Usually reversible.
- Nephrotoxicity and acute infusion reactions are much less common with liposomal amphotericin but still occur
- Arrhythmias, bronchospasm, haematological, rashes, increased LFT's, GI haemorrhage, gastroenteritis, diarrhoea, confusion, encephalopathy, peripheral neuropathy can also occur

Atracurium

Non-depolarising neuro-muscular blocker which is broken down by Hofmann degradation which is dependent on pH and temperature and by ester hydrolysis

Use
- Muscle relaxation

Dose

0.5–0.6 mg/kg bolus

0.1–0.4 mg/kg/h infusion

Side effects

Bradycardia, hypotension

Histamine release

Drug may degrade in the warm atmosphere of PICU

Increased action of metabolite, laudosine in renal and hepatic failure

Atropine

Muscarinic acetylcholine antagonist

Uses
- Sinus bradycardia
- Reversal of muscarinic effects of anticholinesterases
- Organophosphate poisoning
- Drying agent

Dose
15–20 µg/kg IV max 600 µg

Contra-indications/warnings
Pyrexia (increased temperature due to blocking of sweat production)
Urinary retention
Additive effect with other drugs with anti-cholinergic activity, e.g. tri-cyclic anti-depressants

Side effects
Tachycardia
Drowsiness, confusion
Dry mouth
Blurred vision
Atrial arrhythmias and atrioventricular dissociation

Azlocillin
Broad spectrum penicillin

Uses
- systemic infections, respiratory, urinary infection penicillin sensitive streptococci and staphylococci
- anaerobes including Bacteroides
- gram-negative including Pseudomonas

Dose
75 mg/kg IV tds over 1 year
100 mg/kg IV tds 1 month–1 year
100 mg/kg IV bd <1 month (50 mg/kg <2.5 kg)

Contra-indications/warnings
Allergy
Caution with severe jaundice (competitive protein binding)
Reduce dose frequency in renal impairment
Prolongs non-depolarising neuro-muscular blockade

Side effects
Gastrointestinal disturbances
Seizures
Thrombocytopenia

Benzylpenicillin
Bactericidal antibiotic which interferes with bacterial cell wall synthesis

Uses
- meningococcal disease
- neonatal sepsis with gentamicin
- pneumococcal infections

Dose
25 mg/kg IV qds ($\times$ 2–3/day in neonates)
50 mg/kg IV qds or $\times$ 6/day in severe infections, e.g. meningitis

Side effects
Haemolytic anaemia
Transient neutropenia and thrombocytopenia
Convulsions

Contra-indications/warnings
Allergy (use erythromycin or clindamycin)
Anaphylaxis
Renal failure – reduce frequency of administration

Budesonide
Corticosteroid which decreases inflammation and bronchial hypere-activity

Uses
- Asthma prophylaxis
- Mild to moderate croup or post-extubation stridor
- Management of established broncho-pulmonary dysplasia

Dose
Asthma: Nebuliser   250 μg–1 mg bd
                     Up to 2 mg bd over 12
Croup: Nebuliser   2 mg–single dose

Contra-indications
Acute pulmonary tuberculosis
Hypersensitivity

Side effects
Little absorbed into plasma
Occasional mild irritation of throat and hoarseness

Bupivacaine
Use
- Local anaesthetic

Dose
Up to 2 mg/kg bolus
Epidural infusion 0.1–0.2 ml/kg/h of 0.125% solution
Max dose 2 mg/kg per 4 h period
Usually in combination with 1:200 000 epinephrine (adrenaline) for epidural
Can be combined with fentanyl 1 μg/kg

Side effects
Arrhythmias, fits leading to coma
IV injection may lead to fixing of bupivacaine to myocardial tissue and subsequent cardiac arrest

Caffeine citrate
CNS stimulant

Use
• for central apnoea in neonates

Dose
20 mg/kg po/IV loading dose
5 mg/kg od po/IV maintenance dose

Side effects
Jitteriness, seizures, tachycardia

Calcium gluconate
Uses
• Hypocalcaemia
• Cardiac arrest
• Massive transfusion
• Inotrope particularly in neonates and infants

Dose
0.1 ml/kg of 10% solution IV bolus in cardiac arrest
0.1–0.4 ml/kg/h by infusion

Contra-indications/warnings
Hypercalcaemia
Calcium overload is thought to play a role in ischaemic and reperfusion cell injury

Side effects
Local reactions at infusion site including extravasation

Captopril

Angiotensin converting enzyme inhibitor

Use
- hypertension, heart failure

Dose

Commence with test dose as marked hypotension can occur especially if hypovolaemic:

Up to 1 month   10–50 μg/kg

>1 month   100 μg/kg

>12 years   6.25 mg

Maintenance 100 μg/kg–2 mg/kg tds. Titrate to lowest effective dose.

Side effects

Hypotension, GI disturbance, hyperkalaemia, blood disorders

Contra-indications/warnings

Avoid in neonates if possible due to risk of renal failure

Reduce dose in renal failure

Diuretics may potentiate action

NSAIDs reduce hypotensive effect

Cephalosporins

excretion renal

3–7% with penicillin allergy also allergic to cephalosporins

Cefotaxime

Broad spectrum bactericidal

Uses
- meningitis
- initial treatment of severe sepsis including meningococcal disease
- epiglottitis
- respiratory and urinary tract infections

Dose

30–50 mg/kg bd–qds (bd in neonates)

Frequency can be increased in severe infection

Contra-indications/warnings

Allergy to penicillin/cephalosporin

Reduce dosage in renal failure to half at the same frequency

Side effects
Hypersensitivity – rashes
Haematological – can cause neutropenia, thrombocytopenia, haemolytic anaemia, rarely agranulocytosis
Transiently raised LFT's
Pseudomembranous colitis – rare

Ceftazidime
Uses
- third generation cephalosporin
- acts on *Pseudomonas aeruginosa* in particular
- no useful anti-staphylococcal activity

Dose
15–50 mg/kg × 2–3/day; bd in neonates

Contra-indications/warnings
Hypersensitivity
Reduce dose frequency in renal impairment
Care with nephrotoxic drugs (e.g. aminoglycosides, loop diuretics)

Side effects
Pain on injection/phlebitis

Ceftriaxone
Uses
- very similar use and contra-indications as cefotaxime
- third generation cephalosporin

Dose
20–50 mg/kg IV od maximum 4 g
80 mg/kg IV od severe infections

Cefuroxime
Uses
- second generation cephalosporin acts on a wide range of gram-positive and gram-negative bacteria
- lower respiratory tract infections
- surgical prophylaxis

Dose
10–30 mg/kg IV tds (bd <7 days of age)
50–60 mg/kg IV × 3–4/day for meningitis (reduce dose when improvement seen)

Contra-indications/warnings
Hypersensitivity
Renal failure reduce frequency. Removed by haemodialysis.

Side effects
overdose can lead to convulsions
gastrointestinal disturbances

Chloral hydrate
Sedative and hypnotic related to barbiturates

Use
• Sedation usually without respiratory depression. Not analgesic.

Dose
25–50 mg/kg po/pr for single procedures
20–30 mg/kg po/pr up to four times/day

Contra-indications/warnings
Caution in cardiac disease, porphyria, gastritis
Occasionally interacts with IV furosemide to cause sweating, variable blood pressure and a feeling of uneasiness
Hepatic failure may prolong sedation

Side effects
GI irritation
Corrosive to skin
CNS effects: ataxia
Peripheral dilatation leading to hypotension
Myocardial arrhythmias

Cimetidine
H_2-receptor antagonist

Uses
• Prophylaxis against upper GI bleed/perforation, stress ulceration
• Gastro-oesophageal reflux

Dose
5–10 mg/kg   qds
5 mg/kg   qds under 1 month
400 mg/dose qds over 12 months
IV infusion over 10 min

Contra-indications/warnings
Rapid infusion may lead to hypotension and arrhythmias
Reduce dose in renal impairment
Inhibits breakdown of drugs metabolised by cytochrome P450 – warfarin, opiates, phenytoin, theophylline, caffeine

Side effects
Diarrhoea
Headache and tiredness

Ciprofloxacin
A synthetic 4 quinolone antibiotic

Use
• Gram-negative or gram-positive infections

Dose
5 mg/kg bd. Reduce in renal failure. Monitor levels.

Contra-indications
Hypersensitivity
Can reduce threshold of seizures in epilepsy
Patients with glucose-6 dehydrogenase deficiency may be prone to haemolysis

Interactions
May prolong oral anti-coagulants
Reduce theophylline dose
Increased risk of nephrotoxicity with cyclosporin

Side effects
GI disturbances, CNS disturbances, hypersensitivity
Transient hepatic disturbance, also reversible haematological disorders

Clarithromycin
Macrolide antibiotic

Uses
• Respiratory tract infection
• Otitis media

Dose
7.5 mg/kg IV bd max 500 mg/dose

Contra-indications/warning
Hypersensitivity
Interaction with theophylline, digoxin, warfarin, carbamazepine

Side effects
Nausea, vomiting, diarrhoea, abdominal pain
Allergic reactions
Occasional CNS symptoms

Clonidine

α_2 adrenergic agonist. Reduces heart rate, stroke volume and systemic vascular resistance.

Uses
- Sedation
- Morphine withdrawal
- Hypertension

Dose
0.25–5 μg/kg po/IV tds–qds. Need low dose to commence due to possible hypotension.
IV infusion usually 1 μg/kg/h but can go upto 2 μg/kg/h

Contra-indications/warning
Porphyria
Abrupt withdrawal can lead to rebound hypertension

Side effects
Dry mouth, restlessness

Co-trimoxazole

Antibiotic mixture of sulphamethoxazole and trimethoprim

Uses
- *Pneumocystis carinii* pneumonia, toxoplasmosis, urinary tract infections
Dose   18–27 mg/kg IV bd <12 years
         960 mg–1.44 g IV bd 12–18 years
For Pneumocystis: 60 mg/kg IV bd for 14 days then orally for 7 days

Contra-indications
- history of hypersensitivity
- severe renal insufficiency

Side effects
- potentiates warfarin and phenytoin
- rare: Stevens–Johnson syndrome, hepatic necrosis, agranulocytosis, aplastic anaemia
- other haematological side effects are usually reversible
- high dose: rash, fever, raised liver enzymes also can occur

Desmopressin (DDAVP)
Vasopressin analogue

Use
- Diabetes insipidus

Dose

0–1 month	400 ng
1 month–2 years	400 ng–1 µg
2–12	1–2 µg
>12	2–4 µg

Single dose usually suppresses diuresis for 24 h, lower doses may be effective and more gentle

Contra-indications/warnings
Avoid water load
Care with diarrhoea and vomiting
May cause hyponatraemia and convulsions
May interact with tricyclic anti-depressants, chlorpromazine

Dexamethasone
Systemic corticosteroid

Uses
- Improve lung function in broncho-pulmonary dysplasia
- In leukaemia protocols
- Headache with raised intra-cranial pressure
- To reduce oedema around cerebral tumours
- Croup and post-extubation stridor
- Adrenocortical disease
- *Haemophilus meningitis* (may be useful in other causes of meningitis)

Dose
BPD: 500 µg/kg od for 7 days
  250 µg/kg bd for 3 days
Post-extubation stridor 200 µg/kg three doses IV 8 hourly start at least 24 h pre-extubation
Croup 150 µg/kg bd
Headache and raised ICP 250 µg/kg 5 days then reduce

Contra-indications/warnings
Surpresses adrenal for 3–4 weeks after 10 day course
Risk of nephrocalcinosis if on diuretics

May cause hyperglycaemia, muscle weakness, GI haemorrhage, impaired wound healing particularly with prolonged use

Interactions
- Reduced effect with phenobarbitone, phenytoin, rifampicin, carbamazepine
- Antagonises anti-hypertensives and diuretics

Diazepam
Benzodiazepine

Uses
- Sedation
- Anti-convulsant
- Muscle spasms

Dose
0.2 mg/kg bolus IV
0.2–0.5 mg/kg po/pr 8–12 hourly

Contra-indications/warnings
Avoid in neonates as the organic solvents in the intra-venous preparation (propylene glycol and sodium benzoate) are dangerous
Hepatic and renal failure may lead to prolonged effect

Side effects
Pain on injection, thrombophlebitis
Respiratory depression and apnoea
Drowsiness
Hypotension and bradycardia

Diclofenac
Non-steroidal anti-inflammatory analgesic

Uses
- Pain especially musculoskeletal. Has a morphine sparing effect.
- Anti-pyretic

Dose
1 mg/kg tds po/pr max 150 mg/24 h
Can be used by slow IV injection not IM

Contra-indications/warnings
Renal failure
Asthma (especially severe)

GI bleeding or clotting disorders

Hypersensitivity

Not recommended less than 6 months of age

Side effects
Prolongs bleeding time (effect on platelets)

Gastric ulceration, nausea

Acute renal failure particularly if septic, previous poor renal function, hypovolaemia, hypotension

Digoxin
Cardiac glycoside which inhibits Na/K ATPase

Uses
- Supraventricular tachycardia especially by slowing A-V conduction in atrial defibrillation or flutter reducing the ventricular rate. Also positive inotropic effect.
- Congestive cardiac failure

Dose

Age	Digitalisation	Maintenance (given as divided dose)
Premature	20 µg/kg po	5 µg/kg po
Term	30 µg/kg po	8–10 µg/kg po
Child	30–40 µg/kg po	8–12 µg/kg po
>10 years	1500 µg po	125–750 µg po

Digitalisation involves half the dose, then one quarter of the dose 6 h later and the rest 6 h later

Contra-indications/warnings
Complete heart block, in over 2 year olds with an accessory pathway

Reduced doses in renal impairment

Hypokalaemia, hypomagnesaemia and hypercalcaemia may predispose to toxicity

These are potentiated by diuretics, corticosteroids, amphotericin, salbutamol

Plasma concentration of digoxin is increased by anti-arrhythmics including amiodarone, verapamil, diltiazem and also by erythromycin, spironolactone

Side effects
Arrhythmias including heart block

Nausea, vomiting, anorexia, diarrhoea

Fatigue, confusion, hallucinations

Visual disturbances, headache

Dobutamine

A β_1 agonist that increases heart rate and myocardial contractility. Has mild β_2 and α_1 effects reducing peripheral vascular resistance.

Uses
- shock
- sepsis
- cardiomyopathy

Dose
0–20 µg/kg/min

Contra-indications/warnings
- severe hypotension
- obstruction to left ventricular filling or emptying (e.g. subaortic stenosis)
- care when infusing peripherally (dilute)
- ideally infused via central catheter

Side effects
Tachycardia

Dysrhythmias

Nausea, vomiting, hypersensitivity

Tolerance may occur after 72 h

Dopamine

Endogenous catecholamine mainly acting at β_1 and dopaminergic adrenoceptors

Noradrenaline precursor which also releases noradrenaline from synapses

Uses
Inotrope for shock (sepsis)
- low dose (1–5 µg/kg/min) may increase renal blood flow and urine output
- higher dose causes vasoconstriction

Dose
IV infusion of 1–20 µg/kg/min

Contra-indications/warnings
- ventricular tachycardia or other tachyarrhythmias
- phaeochromocytoma
- extravasation may cause tissue irritation and necrosis

D

- variable metabolism means that plasma levels have little relation to infusion rates
- may worsen renal function in a hypovolaemic patient
- interferes with prolactin secretion

Side effects
Tachycardia

Ventricular arrhythmias

Vasoconstriction

Gut ischaemia

Dopexamine
Predominately β_2 stimulating properties
Inodilator with dopaminegric properties

Use
- patients requiring inotropy and peripheral vasodilation, e.g. heart failure

Contra-indications/warnings
Hypertrophic cardiomyopathy

Aortic stenosis

Phaeochromocytoma

Thrombocytopenia may be worsened

Dose
0.5–6 µg/kg/min

Side effects
Tachycardia

Hypotension

Hypokalaemia

Hyperglycaemia

Enoximone
Phosphodiesterase inhibitor

Use
- inotropy with peripheral vasodilation, e.g. in heart failure

Dose
Loading dose 0.5 mg/kg over 1 h
Infusion 5–20 µg/kg/min. No need to wean as it has long half life.

D

Contra-indications/warning
Reduce dose in hepatic or renal failure
Inhibits platelet aggregation

Side effects
Hypotension (especially in septic shock)
Arrhythmias

Epinephrine (Adrenaline)
Direct-acting sympathomimetic activity on α and β adrenoceptors

Uses
- cardiac arrest
- anaphylaxis
- inotrope for sepsis
- croup

Dose
- cardiac arrest – 10 μg/kg IV (100 μg/kg via ETT) 0.1 ml/kg of 1:10 000
- anaphylaxis – IM 0.5–6 years 0.12 ml of 1:1000
                                  6–12 years 0.25 ml of 1:1000
- inotrope 0–2 μg/kg/min via central catheter (may need more)
- nebuliser 0.5 ml/kg up to 5 ml of 1:1000 3 hourly PRN

Contra-indications/warnings
- may cause hyperglycaemia, tachycardia, tremor
- may cause tissue necrosis if extravasasion occurs

Epoprostenol (Prostacyclin)
Prostaglandin which inhibits platelets and is a pulmonary vasodilator

Uses
- Pulmonary vasodilator (inhaled)
- Anti-coagulant (inhibits platelets)
- Digital ischaemia

Dose
IV infusion 2–20 ng/kg/min (via central line on a separate lumen)

Contra-indications/warnings
Hypovolaemia
Potentiates other anti-coagulants

Side effects
Flushing, headaches, hypotension, bradycardia, nausea, convulsions

Erythromycin
Macrolide antibiotic

Uses
- penicillin allergic patients
- active against Streptococcus pneumonia, Group A & B streptococci, Mycoplasma and other atypical pneumonias
- whooping cough. Reduces length of infectivity
- low dose acts as a prokinetic

Dose
12.5 mg/kg qds (tds in neonates)
Dose can be doubled in severe infection

Contra-indications/warnings
Increases serum concentrations of digoxin, warfarin, phenytoin, theophylline, midazolam, alfentanil

Side effects
Nausea, vomiting, diarrhoea, allergy, reversible hearing loss

Fentanyl
Synthetic opioid analgesic – duration of bolus 20 min

Use
- Analgesia

Dose
1–3 μg/kg IV bolus
5–10 μg/kg IV bolus if ventilated
7–10 μg/kg IV bolus to obtund laryngoscopy and intubation
50–100 μg/kg IV bolus for cardiac surgery
1–5 μg/kg/min for sedation
0.5–1 μg/kg/h in epidural with bupivacaine

Side effects
Nausea, constipation, respiratory depression, hypotension, bradycardia
Chest wall rigidity
Enhanced effect in hepatic failure

Flucloxacillin
Antibacterial penicillin

Use
- Gram-positive especially Staphylococcal infections including cellulitis, endocarditis, pneumonia

Dose
12.5–25 mg/kg IV qds (double dose in severe infection)
Reduce frequency in neonates and renal failure

Contra-indications/warnings
Allergy
Prolongs prothrombin time with warfarin

Side effects
Gastrointestinal effects
Skin rash
Hepatitis/cholestatic jaundice

Fluconazole
Triazole antifungal

Uses
- Treatment of fungal infections. Some candida and cryptococcal strains are resistant
- Prophylaxis

Dose
6–12 mg/kg IV/oral od for systemic infection max 400 mg/day
3–12 mg/kg in immunocompromised patients

Contra-indications/warnings
Renal/hepatic impairment

May increase concentrations of warfarin, phenytoin, theophylline and midazolam

Should not be used with cisapride or terfenadine as increased levels may lead to arrhythmias

Side effects
Rash, pruritis
Nausea, vomiting, diarrhoea
Raised liver enzymes (more exaggerated in malignancies or HIV)
Hypersensitivity

Flumazenil
Competitive antagonist to benzodiazepines with short duration of action

Uses
- Benzodiazepine overdose
- Test to diagnose cause of prolonged sedation

Dose
10 µg/kg IV repeated up to a max 40 µg/kg
Infusion 2–10 µg/kg/h

Contra-indications/warnings
Raised ICP
Epilepsy
Tricyclic anti-depressant overdose – may lead to fits and cardiac arrest
Much shorter duration of action than benzodiazepines

Side effects
Dizziness, agitation, fits
Arrhythmias, hypertension
Nausea and vomiting

Furosemide (Frusemide)
Loop diuretic

Use
• diuretic for fluid overload, cardiac or renal failure

Dose
IV 0.5–1 mg/kg od–qds
IV infusion 100 µg–4 mg/kg/h
Suggested start at 100 µg/kg and double every 2 h until urine output
more than 1 ml/kg/h
Higher doses may be required in renal or hepatic failure
Oral doses approximately double IV dose

Contra-indications/warnings
• anuria
• hypokalaemia
• correct hypotension before administration
• precomatose states associated with liver failure
• hypersensitivity
• occasional GI disturbances

Interactions
• may include dysrhythmias in patients on digoxin due to hypokalaemia
• hypotension may occur with ACE inhibitors
• increased risk of ototoxicity with aminoglycosides

Side effects
• electrolyte disturbances: hypokalaemia, hyponatraemia, hypocalcaemia, hypomagnesaemia

- ototoxicity, skin rashes, headache
- acute pancreatitis, bone marrow depression (rare)

Gentamicin
Aminoglycoside antibiotic

Uses
- Septicaemia, bacteraemia, chest infections, neonatal infections
- Intra-thecal for CNS infections

Dose

2.5 mg/kg tds	<12 years
1–2 mg/kg tds	>12 years +
single dose regime	6 mg/kg <12 years
	4–5 mg/kg >12 years

Much reduced in frequency less than 1 month of age
Measurement of trough and peak levels

Contra-indications
Hypersensitivity
Myasthenia gravis
Keep well hydrated and measure renal function

Interactions
Increased risk of oto and nephrotoxicity with cephalosporins, vancomycin, cyclosporin, furosemide, amphotericin
Enhances non-depolarising muscle relaxants

Side effects
Nephrotoxicity. Reduced with once daily dosage.
Ototoxicity

Glyceryl trinitrate
Vasodilator by relaxation of vascular smooth muscle tending to act more on venous than arterial side of the circulation

Uses
- Hypertension
- Increases cardiac output and reduces systemic vascular resistance

Dose
0.2–1 μg/kg/min titrated to effect

Contra-indications/warnings
Hypersensitivity to nitrates
Hypotension, hypovolaemia

Raised ICP

Obstructive cardiomyopathy

Side effects
Hypotension, tachycardia, sweating, headache, nausea, vomiting, restlessness

Heparin
Naturally occurring anti-coagulant which inhibits clotting factors including thrombin by accelerating complexes formed with anti-thrombin III and heparin co-factor II and inactivates factor X

Uses
- Anti-coagulant in extra-corporeal circuits and arterial lines
- Prophylaxis for DVT and pulmonary embolus

Dose
Prophylaxis 75 units/kg calcium heparin s/c

Heparinisation 50–100 units/kg loading dose

IV infusion for embolism   25 units/kg/h <1 year

                                     20 units/kg/h >1 year

Requires monitoring with activated partial thromboplastin time (APTT) 1.5–2.5 × normal

Contra-indications/warnings
Haemorrhagic disorders

GI bleed including peptic ulcer

Recent cerebral haemorrhage

Severe hypertension

Severe liver or renal disease

Post major trauma or surgery

Side effects
Haemorrhage, anaphylactic shock, thrombocytopenia

Skin necrosis

Hydrocortisone
Corticosteroid

Uses
- Anaphylaxis
- Asthma
- *Haemophilus meningitis* (? Other meningitis)

Dose
2.5 mg/kg bolus; 2 mg/kg qds IV <1 month
4 mg/kg bolus; 2–4 mg/kg tds IV 1 month–12 years
100–500 mg bolus then qds >12 years

Contra-indications/warnings
See Dexamethasone

Ibuprofen
Non-steroidal anti-inflammatory analgesic

Uses
• Pain
• Anti-pyretic

Dose
5 mg/kg po qds

Contra-indications/warnings
GI bleeds
Hypersensitivity to aspirin
Care in renal failure/hepatic failure

Side effects
GI disturbance, nausea
Headache, dizziness, vertigo

Ipratropium bromide
Anti-cholinergic bronchodilator

Use
• Acts via parasympathetic nervous system on smooth muscle in lungs. Does seem to be more effective at a younger age than salbutamol nebuliser.

Dose
125 μg <1 year
250 μg <1–5 years
500 μg >5 years
Can be given 2 hourly in severe asthma but usually qds

Contra-indications/side effects
Can occasionally worsen bronchospasm
Atropine like side effects: dry mouth, constipation, urinary retention

Ketamine
Dissociative anaesthetic

Uses
- Analgesia
- Induction of anaesthesia without hypotensive effects

Dose
1–2 mg/kg IV
3–10 mg/kg IM
10–45 µg/kg/min IV infusion for sedation
4 µg/kg/min IV infusion for analgesia

Contra-indications/warnings
Hypertension
Intra-cranial pressure due to increased cerebral blood flow
Pulmonary hypertension

Side effects
Evaluation of blood pressure and heart rate (release of endogenous catecholamines)
Nightmares and hallucinations (reduced by benzodiazepines)
Pain on injection

Labetalol
Combined α and β adrenoceptor antagonist lowers blood pressure by reducing peripheral resistance and blocking the heart from reflex sympathetic stimulation

Use
- Hypertension

Dose
1–2 mg/kg po bd–tds maximum 300 mg
0.5–3 mg/kg/h IV infusion after loading of 0.25–0.5 mg/kg

Contra-indications/warnings
Cardiogenic shock
Heart block
Asthma

Side effects
Bradycardia, hypotension
Heart failure

Lorazepam
Benzodiazepine

Uses
- Sedation
- Anti-convulsant

Dose
0.05–0.1 mg/kg <12 years
4 mg   >12 years

Contra-indications/warnings
Enhances other sedatives or opiates

Side effects
Drowsiness, sedation

Respiratory depression (seems commoner in patients with status epilepticus needing a second dose)

Amnesia

Magnesium sulphate
Uses
- Magnesium supplements
- Hypertension including persistent pulmonary hypertension
- Asthma

Dose
0.2 mmol/kg

Contra-indications/warnings
High levels cause sedation and muscle relaxation
Interaction with non-depolarising muscle relaxants
Rapid IV injection can lead to respiratory or cardiac arrest
Renal impairment leads to high levels

Side effects
Related to serum level
- Nausea and vomiting, slurred speech 4–6.5 mmol/l
- Muscle weakness, respiratory arrest 6.5–7.5 mmol/l
- Cardiac arrest   >10 mmol/l

Mannitol
Osmotic diuretic available as 10% or 20%

Uses
- Raised intra-cranial pressure if serum osmolality <300 mosm/l

- Oedema including ascites
- Prevention of renal failure in jaundiced patients

Dose
250 mg–1.5 g/kg. Max 2 g/kg/day IV.

Contra-indications
Inadequate urine flow
Pulmonary oedema or congestive heart failure
Dehydration or acidosis
Intra-cranial bleeding (relative)

Interactions
Oral anti-coagulants may have reduced effect
Hypokalaemia may lead to digoxin toxicity

Side effects
Fluid and electrolyte imbalance
Pulmonary oedema
CNS toxicity with overdose

Meropenem
Carbapenem β-lactam antibiotic

Uses
- very broad spectrum – gram-positive and gram-negative including anaerobes
- inactive against methicillin resistant staphylococcus aureus (MRSA)
- reserved for infections resistant to other antibiotics

Dose
20 mg/kg IV tds for pneumonia, peritonitis, septicaemia
40 mg/kg IV tds for meningitis and life threatening infections

Contra-indications/warnings
Allergy
Renal failure reduce dose frequency; removed by haemodialysis
Care in patients with liver disease

Side effects
Thrombophlebitis, skin rashes, gastrointestinal upset, raised LFT's, pseudomembranous colitis rarely, reversible haematological features – neutropenia

Metronidazole
Antimicrobial

Use
- anaerobic bacterial and protozoal infections

Dose
7.5 mg/kg IV tds (bd in neonates)

Contra-indications
Care in renal and hepatic failure, potentiates warfarin, phenytoin, alcohol

Side effects
Nausea, vomiting, GI disturbances, darkening of urine, drowsiness, dizziness, headache, ataxia, seizures (rarely)

Midazolam
Water soluble benzodiazepine

Uses
- Sedation and anxiolysis
- Anti-convulsant

Dose
Bolus 50–100 µg/kg/min
Intra-venous infusion 120–360 µg/kg/min

Contra-indications/warnings
- Can accumulate leading to prolonged sedation
- Abrupt withdrawal can lead to an acute withdrawal syndrome therefore reduce infusion slowly
- Care in patients with hepatic and renal dysfunction

Side effects
Oversedation
Hypotension
Respiratory depression
Enhanced effects in hepatic failure

Interactions
Midazolam is metabolised by cytochrome P450 in the liver and therefore is affected by enzyme inducers and inhibitors. Therefore effects are increased by erythromycin, cimetidine, metronidazole and fluconazole.

Milrinone
Selective phosphodiesterase inhibitor

Use
- Congestive cardiac failure. Increases cardiac output, reducing systemic

vascular resistance and pulmonary capillary wedge pressure. Does not increase heart rate.

Dose
50 µg/kg loading dose over 10 min then
0.375–0.75 µg/kg/min

Contra-indications/warnings
Atrial flutter or fibrillation – may increase ventricular rate
Reduce dose in renal failure

Side effects
Hypotension
Arrhythmias

Morphine
Opiate analgesic

Use
• Analgesia and sedation

Dose
0.1–0.2 mg/kg IV bolus
10–80 µg/kg/h IV infusion if ventilated
Reduce dose in neonates and infants and if not ventilated. Titrate to response.

Contra-indications/warnings
Care in patients with respiratory depression, raised intra-cranial pressure or head injury if not ventilated
Liver and renal impairment

Side effects
Nausea and vomiting, ileus, biliary spasm
Hypotension
Increased susceptibility to respiratory depression in neonates

Naloxone
Opioid antagonist. Duration of action 30–45 min.

Use
• Reversal of opioid effects of respiratory depression, sedation, urinary retention, pruritus

Dose
10 µg/kg IV if unsuccessful 100 µg/kg (max 2 mg)
Infusion 5–20 µg/kg/h
Titrate dose if post-operative to avoid sudden pain

Contra-indications/warning
Post-operatively leading to pain, haemodynamic disturbance

Side effects
Arrhythmias, hypertension

Norepinephrine (Noradrenaline)
α adrenoceptor mediated vasoconstrictor

Use
• Vasoconstriction in sepsis 'warm shock'

Dose
0–2 µg/kg/min via central catheter

Contra-indications/warnings
Normovolaemia

Extravasation

Side effects
Hypertension with bradycardia

Headache

Peripheral gangrene

Nystatin
Antifungal

Use
• Prevention and treatment of candida infection

Dose
1 ml qds orally

Side effects
Nausea, vomiting, diarrhoea rarely rashes

Ondansetron
5HT$_3$ antagonist

Use
• Post-operative and chemotherapy induced anti–emetic

Dose
0.1 mg/kg IV slowly tds max 8 mg

Side effects
Headaches, flushing, constipation
Care in hepatic failure (increases liver enzymes)

Pancuronium
Non-depolarising necromuscular blockade with medium duration of action (40 min plus). Causes increase in blood pressure and heart rate.

Use
- Muscle relaxation

Dose
0.1 mg/kg bolus
0.1 mg/kg/h infusion

Side effects
Hypertension and tachycardia
Prolonged paralysis in hepatic or renal failure
Effects prolonged by aminoglycosides, magnesium, clindamycin, propranolol

Paracetamol
Analgesic and anti-pyretic

Uses
- Mild pain
- Anti-pyretic

Dose
10–30 mg/kg/dose po max total 90 mg/kg/day for 48 h
Max up to 3 months of age 60 mg/kg/day
4–6 hourly po/pr. Larger doses are required rectally.
IV (propacetamol) 30 mg/kg qds

Contra-indications/warnings
Risk of hepatic damage with overdose

Phenobarbitone
Barbiturate

Use
- Epilepsy

Dose
15 mg/kg IV loading dose (up to 20 mg/kg in neonates)
2.5–5 mg/kg IV bd maintenance

Contra-indications/warnings
Reduce dose and measure levels in renal/hepatic disease
Enzyme inducer reducing effect of many anti-epileptics

Side effects
Sedation, ataxia, respiratory depression

Phenytoin
Anti-epileptic

Uses
- Epilepsy
- Anti-arrhythmic especially for digoxin toxicity

Dose
18 mg/kg IV loading dose >1 month
2.5–7.5 mg/kg po bd maintenance

Contra-indications/warnings
Rapid IV administration (severe hypotension or CNS depression)
Severe liver disease (reduce dose)
Measure serum levels
Numerous drug reactions as phenytoin is an enzyme inducer

Side effects
Nystagmus, ataxia, slurred speech
Drowsiness and confusion
Rashes
Inducing haematological effects due to folate deficiency
Gum hypertrophy

Piperacillin
Tazocin includes piperacillin and tazobactam which is active against
β-lactamase producing bacteria resistant to penicillin

Uses
- Pseudomonas infections
- Also gram-negative bacilli including Proteus sp and B fragilis

Dose
50–75 mg IV qds in severe infection. Max 4 g/day.
50–100 mg IV tds in neonates

Contra-indications
Allergy to penicillin
May interact with warfarin and neuro-muscular blocking agents

Side effects
Rare severe anaphylaxis
Liver disorders, blood dyscrasias, skin rashes

Promethazine
Phenothiazine with anti-histamine and sedative effects

Use
• Sedation

Dose
1–2 mg/kg single dose
0.5–1 mg/kg qds

Contra-indications/warnings
Avoid in neonates and premature infants

Side effects
Occasionally irritable or excitable behaviour
Dizziness, restlessness, headaches, extrapyramidal effects
Hypotension, tachycardia

Propofol
Induction agent for general anaesthesia

Uses
• General anaesthesia
• Sedation

Dose
Up to 3.5 mg/kg. Titrate dose to effect as younger and less ill children will need more.
Infusion 4–12 mg/kg/h but not recommended for long-term use in those aged under 16.

Contra-indications/warnings
Care in patients with hypovolaemia, epilepsy, severe cardiac or respiratory disease

Side effects
Pain on injection
Hypotension, bradycardia
Apnoea
Convulsions
Fat overload

Has been implicated in propofol infusion syndrome which has led to fatalities due to cerebral problems associated with hyperlipidaemia and metabolic acidosis, mostly associated with children with upper respiratory tract infections.

Prostaglandin E1 (Alprostadil)

Use
- Maintenance of patent ductus arteriosus in duct-dependent cardiac disease

Dose
0.01–0.1 μg/kg/min IV infusion
Titrated up to 0.4 μg/kg/min

Side effects
Apnoea, usually transient
Seizures, fever, diarrhoea
Flushing, bradycardia, hypotension

Protamine

Basic protein which has anti-coagulant effect

Use
- Combines with acidic heparin to neutralise the effect of heparin

Dose
1 ml of 1% (10 mg) will neutralise 1000 units of heparin given 15 min before. 1 ml per 25 ml of pumped blood. Give as slow bolus.

Side effects
- Rapid bolus leads to pulmonary vasoconstriction, reduced left arterial pressure and hypotension
- Flushing, headache, dyspnoea, hypotension

Ranitidine

H_2 receptor antagonist

Use
- Prophylaxis against bleeding from GI tract

Dose
1 mg/kg tds   up to 6 months
125–250 μg/kg/h   continuous infusion
Can be added to TPN

Contra-indications/warnings
May mask other gastric diseases

Side effects
Hypersensitivity can vary from urticaria to anaphylactic shock
Rarely acute pancreatitis, leucopenia, thrombocytopenia
Bradycardia and AV block particularly if given rapidly IV
Transient rise in liver function tests

Salbutamol
β_2 agonist

Uses
- Bronchodilation
- Reduces hyperkalaemia
- Vasodilator

Dose

Nebuliser	2.5–5 mg	(1.25–2.5 mg under 1 month)

Can be repeated up to half-hourly for asthma or single dose for hyper-kalaemia

IV	15 µg/kg	for status asthmaticus initially
IV infusion	1–5 µg/kg/min	for status asthmaticus or as a vasodilator
IV bolus	4 µg/kg	hyperkalaemia

Contra-indications/warnings
Increased risk of hypokalaemia especially with high dose cortico-steroids, diuretics, theophylline
Has caused ketoacidosis in diabetics

Side effects
Usually dose related and more frequent with systemic therapy: hypokalaemia, tremor, nervousness, tachycardia

Sodium bicarbonate
Uses
- Metabolic acidosis
- May be needed in renal replacement therapy
- Cardiac arrest

Dose
$1/3 \times$ base deficit $\times$ weight = ml 8.4% sodium bicarbonate
Half this dose is given to assess response
In neonates and small infants use 4.2% to reduce the osmolarity

Contra-indications/warnings
Do not give with other drugs especially calcium or inotropes
Hypokalaemia may be worsened

Side effects

Metabolic alkalosis

Extravasation (give centrally if possible)

Fluid load

Sodium nitroprusside

Vasodilator reducing both preload and afterload by direct action on vascular smooth muscle particularly on the arterial side of the circulation

Use

• Hypertension

Dose

0.5–8 µg/kg/min IV titrated to response

Contra-indications/warnings

Severe hepatic impairment

Protect from light

Side effects

Headache, dizziness, nausea, palpitations, apprehension, sweating

Reflex tachycardia

Methaemoglobinaemia

Acute withdrawal can cause hypertensive crisis

Spironolactone

Aldosterone antagonist, potassium sparing diuretic

Use

• Cardiac failure, ascites, potentiation of other diuretics

Dose

750 µg–1.5 mg/kg po bd   <12 years

25–50 mg   >12 years

or IV as potassium canrenoate 1–2 mg/kg bd

Dose conversion: oral spironolactone: IV potassium canrenoate 0.7:1

Contra-indications/warnings

Severe renal impairment, hyperkalaemia, Addison's disease

Hyponatraemia

Can worsen potential of other drugs to produce hyperkalaemia

May falsely increase digoxin levels

Side effects
Renal function deterioration, hyperkalaemia, hyponatraemia, GI disturbances, drowsiness, headache, skin rashes

Sucralfate
Mucosal protector

Use
- Prevention and treatment of stress ulceration

Dose

1 month–2 years	250 mg	4–6/day
2–12	500 mg	4–6/day
>12	1 g	4–6/day

Contra-indications/warnings
Hypersensitivity
Caution with children with renal impairment due to aluminium absorption
May reduce oral bio-availability of digoxin, warfarin, phenytoin, ciprofloxacin
Avoid antacids within half an hour
Avoid enteral feeds within 1 h

Side effects
Hypersensitivity – pruritus, oedema and urticaria, constipation, nausea, vomiting, diarrhoea, headache, dizziness, drowsiness
Hyperphosphataemia especially in patients with renal failure

Suxamethonium
Depolarising neuro-muscular blocker. Rapid onset and short duration.

Use
- Rapid intubation of trachea
- Management of severe post-extubation laryngospasm

Dose
1–1.5 mg/kg IV for intubation. Need atropine for bradycardia with second dose.

Contra-indications/warnings
Hyperkalaemia
Risk of exaggerated rise in potassium may occur:
  – Severe burns
  – Muscle damage

- Paraplegia and quadraplegia
- Peripheral neuropathy, e.g. Guillain-Barre
- Congenital myopathies
- Disuse atrophy

History of malignant hyperpyrexia

Myasthenia gravis (resistance)

Side effects

Muscle pain

Bradycardia (especially after second dose)

Hyperkalaemia

Malignant hyperpyrexia trigger

Increase intra-ocular and intra-cranial pressures

Prolonged apnoea with pseudocholinesterase deficiency

Teicoplanin

Glycopeptide antibiotic

Uses

- Serious gram-positive infections
- Can be used for treatment of infected implanted lines as a lock

Dose

<1 month	16 mg/kg od loading dose
	8 mg/kg od maintenance
>1 month	10 mg/kg bd for 3 doses
	10 mg/kg od maintenance

Contra-indications/warnings

Hypersensitivity

Care with ototoxic and nephrotoxic drugs

Side effects

Irritation on injection

Transient increase in serum creatinine and liver enzymes

Thrombocytopenia and other blood dyscrasias (rare)

Rarely causes ototoxicity or nephrotoxicity

Thiopentone

Barbiturate whose action is terminated by redistribution. Therefore repeated doses cause accumulation.

Uses

- Induction of anaesthesia
- Status epilepticus

T

Dose
2–5 mg IV bolus. May need more in well children
2–8 mg/kg/h IV infusion

Contra-indications/warnings
Avoid in porphyria
Hypovolaemia

Side effects
Induces enzymes
Hypotension especially if hypovolaemic
Myocardial depression
Respiratory depression
Hypersensitivity reactions (rare but serious), histamine release
Tissue necrosis from extravasation (alkaline solution)
Intra-arterial injection can lead to limb necrosis

Trimeprazine
Phenothiazine derivative

Use
• Sedation

Dose
2 mg/kg po up to 90 mg maximum tds

Contra-indications/warnings
Avoid in hepatic or renal dysfunction
Epilepsy, hypothyroidism

Side effects
Excitability, dry mouth

Vancomycin
A glycopeptide antibiotic

Uses
• Active against gram-positive bacteria. Used for severe life-threatening infections which other drugs have not treated successfully including MRSA.
• Pseudomembranous colitis

Dose
15 mg/kg loading dose
10 mg/kg maintenance qds
>12 years 500 mg qds max 2 g/24 h

Contra-indications/warnings
Care in renal failure (measure levels)

Hypersensitivity

May potentiate other nephrotoxic drugs including aminoglycosides, amphotericin

Side effects
Nephrotoxicity

Ototoxicity

Reversible haematological disorders

Vecuronium

Non-depolarising muscle relaxant. It has no cardiovascular effects. Duration of action 20–30 min.

Use
• Muscle relaxation

Dose
0.1 mg/kg IV bolus

0.1 mg/kg/h infusion

Side effects
May be prolonged in hepatic or renal failure

BIBLIOGRAPHY

Advanced Life Support Group. Advanced Paediatric Life Support. The Practical Approach. Third edition. London: BMJ Books, 2001.

Duncan A. Paediatric Intensive Care. London: BMJ Books, 1998.

Fuhrman BP, Zimmermann JJ. Pediatric Critical Care. Second edition. St Louis: Mosby, 1998.

McConachie Z. Handbook of ICU Therapy. London: Greenwich Medical Media, 1999.

Paediatric Intensive Care Society. Standards of Bereavement Care. Sheffield: PICS, 2002.

Pearson G. Handbook of Paediatric Intensive Care. London: WB Saunders, 2002.

RCPCH Medicines for Children. London: RCPCH, 1999.

Rogers MC, Helfaer MA. Handbook of Pediatric Intensive Care. Third edition. Baltimore: Williams and Wilkins, 1999.

Index

References to drug descriptions in Section 3 are highlighted in italics.

INDEX

INDEX

INDEX

INDEX

INDEX

INDEX

INDEX